GOING UNIVERSAL

GOING UNIVERSAL

How 24 Developing Countries Are Implementing Universal Health Coverage Reforms from the Bottom Up

Daniel Cotlear, Somil Nagpal, Owen Smith,
Ajay Tandon, and Rafael Cortez

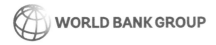 **WORLD BANK GROUP**

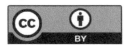

Contents

Boxes

Figures

Foreword

When World Bank Group President Jim Yong Kim addressed the 66th session of the World Health Assembly in May 2013[1], he called for the global community to "bend the arc of history to ensure that everyone in the world has access to affordable, quality health services in a generation."

President Kim's clarion call echoes the World Bank's aim in health, nutrition and population: To accelerate progress toward universal health coverage (UHC)—ensuring that by 2030 everyone has access to essential, quality health care, regardless of their ability to pay. Recent World Health Organization and World Bank Group estimates[2] show us that despite the great progress countries have made on the path to UHC, we still have far to go: 400 million people lack access to essential health services, and 6 percent of people in developing countries are tipped into or pushed further into extreme poverty because of health spending.

UHC is a triple win: It improves people's health, reduces poverty, and fuels economic growth. That's why the Health, Nutrition and Population Global Practice is working with governments, the private sector, and civil society, as well as with other development partners, to: establish systems for fair, efficient, and sustainable financing of health; scale up and strengthen front-line and facility-based services; and harness the potential of other sectors that contribute to health, nutrition, and population outcomes. In working in these areas, we are sourcing the best evidence globally to support appropriate choice and effective implementation of solutions, according to context.

Going Universal: How 24 Developing Countries are Implementing Universal Health Coverage Reforms from the Bottom Up is an important contribution to this global evidence base. The book is about 24 developing countries that have embarked on the long journey toward UHC and are following a "bottom-up" approach to embrace the least well-off, even at the start of that journey. Each UHC program analyzed is seeking to overcome the legacy of inequality by tackling both a financing gap and a provision gap—because UHC requires not just more money but also a shift in spending. The book will help policy makers understand the options they face and help develop a new operational research agenda.

Most of these UHC programs are less than a decade old; together, they cover one third of the world's population. They are also transformational in their efforts to improve the way health systems operate, offering the potential to achieve greater equity and better results for the money spent. The report identifies key risks that lie ahead and identifies an emerging agenda where more country and global learning is required.

The report offers those committed to the achievement of UHC worldwide a valuable new resource to help chart evidence and experience-informed pathways toward accelerated progress.

Dr. Timothy Evans
Senior Director, Health, Nutrition and Population
World Bank Group

Notes

1. http://www.worldbank.org/en/news/speech/2013/05/21/world-bank -group-president-jim-yong-kim-speech-at-world-health-assembly.
2. http://www.who.int/healthinfo/universal_health_coverage/report/2015/en/.

About the Authors

Daniel Cotlear was the team leader for the program that produced the 24 country studies on which this book is based and for the production of the book. He is Lead Economist at the World Bank's Global Practice on Health, Nutrition, and Population, with a focus on developing tools to support countries in the implementation of universal health coverage. He has been involved in the preparation of dozens of country studies and of many policy and investment projects in three continents. Before joining the Bank he taught economics and was advisor to the Ministry of Agriculture of Peru.

Somil Nagpal is a New Delhi–based Senior Health Specialist with the World Bank's Global Practice on Health, Nutrition, and Population, and works on health financing, health systems, and universal health coverage in several countries in Asia. Before joining the World Bank in 2009, he worked with India's federal insurance regulator and led the Health department therein. He has also worked with the Indian ministries of health and finance, India's commission on Macroeconomics and Health, and the World Health Organization.

Owen Smith is a Senior Economist in the Health, Nutrition, and Population Global Practice of the World Bank, where he has worked on health financing, health policy, and other human development issues in the Europe and Central Asia and South Asia regions. Before joining the World Bank in 2005, he worked as a health economist with Abt Associates and as a country economist at the Canadian Ministry of Finance.

Ajay Tandon is a Washington, DC–based Senior Economist with the World Bank's Global Practice on Health, Nutrition, and Population, where he works on a variety of issues related to health financing, fiscal space, service delivery, and universal health coverage. Before joining the World Bank in 2007, he worked with the Asian Development Bank and with the Evidence and Information for Policy department of the World Health Organization.

Rafael Cortez is a Senior Economist at the World Bank's Health, Nutrition, and Population Global Practice. He has worked in the design and management of health sector projects in Bank client countries, and in health financing and population economics issues. Before joining the World Bank, he worked as a Professor in Economics with the Universidad del Pacífico, and as an economics advisor at the Peruvian National Health Insurance Agency.

Acknowledgments

This book has been prepared by a team led by Daniel Cotlear and comprising Somil Nagpal, Owen Smith, Ajay Tandon, and Rafael Cortez. Research assistance and many good ideas were provided by Anooj Pattnaik and Hui Wang for the preparation of the book. Sarah McCune assisted the team during the data-collection period during which the country case studies were prepared. Jonathan Cavanagh copy-edited the first draft of the book. After that, the book underwent many changes and Jonathan Aspin worked with the team to produce the final drafts.

The team wishes to express special thanks to Nicole Klingen, for facilitating and encouraging their work, and to the following peer reviewers who generously spent time and effort helping in the design of the research project and in commenting on several drafts of the manuscript: Joe Kutzin, Adam Wagstaff, Ricardo Bitran, Marcelo Giugale, Christoph Kurowski, and Michele Gragnolati. Valuable contributions and general guidance at various stages of the project were provided by Tim Evans, Olusoji O. Adeyi, Cristian Baeza, Enis Barış, Daniel Dulitzky, Leslie K. Elder, Armin Fidler, Ariel Fiszbein, Joana Godhino, Trina S. Haque, Beth King, Akiko Maeda, Julie McLaughlin, Toomas Palu, and Abdo Yazbeck.

This book synthesizes 24 developing-country case studies and two wider reviews of evidence and the literature—together, the "UNICO studies" (Appendix 1). The authors were: Nelly Aguilera, Eduardo Alfonso, Chokri Arfa, Chris Atim, Oscar Bernal, Aarushi Bhatnagar, Ricardo Bitran, Maria Eugenia Bonilla-Chacin, Sarbani Chakraborty, Shiyan Chao, Rafael Cortez, Elina M. Dale, Yadira Diaz, Huong Lan Dao, Tania Dmytraczenko, Heba Elgazzar, Pedro Franke, Ursula Giedion, Antonio Giuffrida, Piya Hanvoravongchai, Pandu Harimurti, Melitta Jakab, Robert Janett, Hannah Kikaya, Jack Langenbrunner, Lilin Liang, Rekha Menon, Somil Nagpal, Patrick Osewe, Eko Pambudi, Christine Lao Pena, Anna Pigazzini, Gandham N.V. Ramana, Daniela Romero,

Karima Saleh, Owen Smith, Aparnaa Somanathan, Ajay Tandon, Tran Van Tien, Fernando Montenegro Torres, Netsanet Workie.

In addition to the people listed above, many people both inside and outside the World Bank helped with the book. In particular, valuable comments were received from World Bank staff and consultants, including: Helene Barroy, Hortenzia Beciu, Paolo Belli, Mukesh Chawla, Joy Antoinette De Beyer, Jean J. De St Antoine, Francois Diop, Maria Luisa Escobar, Ashley Fox, Ursula Gideon, Pablo Gottret, Charles C. Griffin, Margaret Grosh, Alaa Mahmoud Hamed, Gerard La Forgia, Maureen Lewis, Rong Li, James Christopher Lovelace, Gayle Martin, Andre Medici, Ha Thi Hong Nguyen, Robert Oelrichs, Philip O'Keefe, Robert J. Palacios, Brian Pascual, Alex Preker, George Schieber, Meera Shekar, Edit Velenyi, Monique Vledder, Wei Aun Yap, and Elif Yavuz.

Those outside the World Bank who contributed substantially with comments and material included: Margaret Cornelius and Dan Kress (Bill & Melinda Gates Foundation), Amanda Glassman (Center for Global Development), Rifat Atun, Peter Berman, Margaret Kruk and Michael Reich (Harvard University), Juan Pablo Uribe (Fundacion Colombia), Viroj Tangcharoensathien (International Health Policy Program), Octavio Gómez-Dantés (National Institute of Public Health, Mexico), Anne Mills (London School of Hygiene & Tropical Medicine), Robert Marten, Stefan Nachuk and Jeanette Vega (Rockefeller Foundation), Karen Cavanaugh and Ariel Pablos-Méndez (USAID), Cheryl Cashin, Amanda Folsom, David De Ferranti, Robert Hecht, and Gina Lagomarsino (Results for Development), Michael Adelhardt (P4H), and David Evans, and Inke Mathauer (World Health Organization).

The project could not have been undertaken without the financial cooperation of the Bill & Melinda Gates Foundation, whose assistance is warmly acknowledged.

Abbreviations

CHW	Community health worker
GDP	Gross domestic product
MoH	Ministry of Health
MDG	Millennium Development Goal
ISP	Informal sector program
OECD	Organisation for Economic Co-operation and Development
OOPE	Out-of-pocket expenditure
PVP	Poor and vulnerable program
SHI	Social health insurance
SHI+	Poor and vulnerable program embedded in SHI
SHI++	Informal sector program embedded in SHI
SSP	Supply-side program
TR	Targeting registry
UHC	Universal health coverage
UNICO	Universal Health Coverage Studies Series
WHO	World Health Organization

A list of abbreviations for individual country UHC programs can be found in Table 1.1, page 26.

Overview

Introduction—Chapter 1

This book is about 24 developing countries that have embarked on the long journey toward universal health coverage (UHC) following a bottom-up approach, with a special focus on the poor and vulnerable. The main objective of the book is to describe these countries' experiences based on a systematic data collection effort that sought to capture in great detail *how* they are implementing UHC. Drawing on global experience, the book aims to provide practical insights to policy makers and others who seek to accelerate progress toward UHC worldwide.

The 24 countries were selected for their significant efforts of the past decade or so to expand coverage of health care services while keeping a special focus on the poor and having the overarching objective of attaining UHC. While these countries do not constitute an exhaustive list of all UHC reforms around the world today, together they cover over one-third of the world's population, and therefore offer an important data set from which to learn about UHC worldwide and, more specifically, about the bottom-up approach to UHC.

The starting point for bottom-up UHC programs is, in a single word, *inequality*—all too often the poor get much less from their health systems than the better off. Health systems are unequal in many different ways. The poor are often in a different subsystem with less funding per person. They may not have access to the same providers as the rich, and get substandard care as a result. The poor often cannot pay for even small costs of care if they are not covered, such as for drugs or medical supplies that are out of stock, or those for transport to reach the nearest health facility. These costs can be an insurmountable deterrent for them. When there is "implicit rationing" (often related to issues like limited presence of providers, patchy geographic access, crowding at facilities, and quantitative restrictions), the rich can often use their connections (or money) to jump the queue. The poor may live in rural areas where good care is hard to find. Or public spending may be heavily concentrated on a tertiary hospital in the capital city. The poor may also belong to historically disadvantaged groups, such as ethnic minorities, who face discrimination when they seek care. The list could go on ...

Each of the UHC programs analyzed in this book is seeking to overcome the legacy of inequality by tackling both a "financing gap" and a "provision gap": the financing gap (or lower per capita spending on the poor) by spending additional resources in a pro-poor way; the provision gap (or underperformance of service delivery for the poor) by expanding supply and changing incentives in a variety of ways. Thus most UHC policy makers appear to have converged around a view that the road to UHC will require not just more money but also a laser-like focus on changing the rules of the game for spending health system resources.

The 24 countries are adopting two broad approaches to bottom-up UHC, as the 26 programs show (India has three programs in the study). The first, referred to here as "supply-side programs," channels investments to expand the capacity of service provision through more funding for inputs (for example, human resources) and for reforms such as greater flexibility in staff recruitment, financial autonomy for public clinics, strong organizational protocols, and explicit performance indicators. There are eight such programs in our sample. They are "bottom up" because they focus on the services typically used by the poor—in six out of the eight, the focus is on primary health care, often with an emphasis on rural areas, where supply capacity is frequently lacking.

The second broad approach encompasses "demand-side programs." These programs attach resources to an identified population and the services they use. They often do this by identifying and enrolling their target population and purchasing health care services on their behalf via output-based payments. The 18 programs following this approach can be further divided into four groups according to which subpopulations are covered and how (chapter 1, table 1.2).

The discussion of this book is largely descriptive, not prescriptive—it does not attempt to identify "best practice," for example. But the book aims to help policy makers understand the options they face, and to help develop a new operational research agenda based on a deeper understanding of what challenges policy makers are facing. While the main chapters of the book are focused on providing a granular understanding of policy design, appendix C shows the results of a systematic review of the literature on impact evaluation. This exercise identified over 6,500 studies attempting to evaluate UHC program impact on access to services, on financial protection, and on health outcomes. Despite the success of individual studies to stir debate leading to program adjustments in the countries studied, overall this literature is not very useful as a *guide* for policy makers facing the next generation of UHC reform challenges because in the aggregate the results are inconclusive and do not tell us *why* some programs have an impact—and others do not. The main limitation comes from comparing "apples and pears": the individual studies measure the impact of a certain program, but do not identify the necessary design feature of the program to allow for controlled comparisons. In this book we show that each UHC program involves several components, that each component requires choices, and that the quality of implementation of the individual components matters. If a program does not have an impact, the existing methodology is incapable of identifying which component of the program is "not working." A new generation of operational research therefore will need to unbundle programs into their key components and examine if each component "works" separately. A first step to design the new research agenda is to provide a granular understanding of program design; that is what this book provides.

The book analyzes dozens of policy decisions at country level that shed light on how UHC programs are implemented in countries around the world, for which appendix B offers some background. The data-collection tool for the analysis comprised a common "Nuts & Bolts" questionnaire with nine modules (appendix D). Its modules collected information on a country's health system, detailing information on the UHC program. The unit of analysis is the UHC program, not the entire health system, although much contextual information on the latter was collected. This program approach is used to focus on what is new or changing, because this is where reforms are concentrated. While this approach may run the risk of losing sight of the "system" once we dive into the details of a program, its advantage is that it allows for a much deeper understanding of how nascent UHC programs are functioning—and changing. In addition, the UHC programs are often serving to leverage broader reform of the health system, in effect blurring the distinction between program and system.

The rest of this overview follows the organizing framework for the book: after an introduction in chapter 1, chapters 2 through 6 present the main findings. Each focuses on a core set of policies and identifies key trends and implications within each set. Chapters 2, 3, and 4 correspond roughly to the three dimensions of the "UHC cube" popularized by the World Health Organization: people, benefits, and money. Chapter 5, on improving health care provision, builds on chapter 3 (benefits) to look at service delivery. Chapter 6, on accountability, looks at how stated objectives within each of the other topics are met and ensured. Chapter 7 summarizes the key chapter messages and draws out implications for the UHC agenda. (The appendixes have been touched on above.)

Covering People—Chapter 2

Achieving UHC is, first and foremost, about covering people. It is individuals and households who suffer the consequences of poor access to health care services and a high financial burden when they actually seek care. The framework for the book's analysis recognizes that populations in developing countries are typically segmented into three broad subpopulations: the poor and vulnerable, the nonpoor informal sector, and the formal sector. In many countries each population is covered differently by the health system. Countries that employ a bottom-up approach acknowledge this segmentation and have developed strategies to reach each subpopulation, such as targeting to ensure that the poor and vulnerable are not left behind.

Key Trends

Countries may use supply- or demand-side programs to strengthen coverage for lower-income populations. In most countries, these populations are initially covered by the Ministry of Health (MoH). Supply-side programs aim to reform and upgrade the production of health care services, prioritizing the poor and vulnerable through geographic targeting and an emphasis on primary care and on the services that they often use; demand-side programs aim to reduce the economic barriers for prioritized subpopulations, expanding their access to more and better services, with wider choice of providers and modalities to improve financial protection.

Many demand-side programs use personal identification systems that "give a face to the poor," and that rely on increasingly complex mechanisms of targeting, usually entailing a shift from simple systems to more precise systems managed by a "targeting registry," which is often linked to the central government's ministry in charge of social assistance. Targeting approaches allow for a prioritization of health budgets for the poor, but they also incur significant administrative costs and may encounter political challenges from those who do not benefit.

Demand-side programs often involve several phases during which additional subpopulations are sequentially enrolled. These programs' typical initial mandate is to enroll the poor and vulnerable, later entering a second phase with an expanded mandate to include the nonpoor informal sector. The participation of the poor is always tax financed, but this second-phase expansion can take two paths: contributory and noncontributory.

The contributory path often involves embedding the program within the agency for social health insurance (SHI). Those in the nonpoor informal sector can often initially join the SHI program by making voluntary contributions, and over time as the capacity to enforce the payment of contributions from this group improves, its participation becomes de facto mandatory (as in Chile, for example).

Countries following the noncontributory path typically create programs that operate autonomously from SHI agencies, financing these programs via taxes. Countries with an SHI system have pros and cons when enrolling those in the nonpoor informal sector via the noncontributory path. An advantage is that the expansion of coverage from the poor to the rest of the informal sector can be very rapid; a disadvantage is the emergence of a trade-off between equity in the benefit package (comparing the autonomous program and the SHI) and fiscal sustainability (due to higher costs and the potential increase in informality). Resolving this trade-off may require deep tax and health-system reforms to replace the dual SHI/MoH system with a fully tax-funded system. Enrolling those in the nonpoor informal sector through a contributory path presents fewer risks for sustainability but also entails a slower pace in expanding coverage, as it requires development of capacities to identify incomes and to collect contributions from beneficiaries in the sector.

There is abundant evidence that voluntary insurance is not a viable path to UHC. It is, however, a useful stepping stone—a transitional phase that serves certain objectives while countries develop the capacity to establish either a mandatory contributory system or the capacity to pay for a noncontributory tax-financed system. The usefulness of voluntary insurance is partly to provide financial protection to a small, but often influential and vocal, sliver of the population. In the realm of political economy, it gives countries the opportunity to begin the process of expansion of coverage of the poor and vulnerable.

While tax-financed coverage of the poor and vulnerable can be achieved by low- and middle-income countries, expansion to cover the rest of the informal sector is more demanding of fiscal revenues and implementation capacity, and has been easier to achieve in richer countries as they have smaller informal sectors, lower poverty rates, greater government revenues, and stronger institutions. These "socioeconomic fundamentals" determine a country's ability to cover its nonpoor informal sector.

Policy Implications

- *The bottom-up approach is a viable option for developing countries.* Countries interested in pursuing a progressive path to expand health coverage may wish to consider this approach.

- *Prioritizing the poor and vulnerable within a bottom-up approach may require identification and targeting capacities to be developed.* As countries improve the benefits, quality, and financial protection of publicly financed health care they can no longer rely on traditional systems of implicit targeting (the better off opting out from the unattractive public services) and must develop the capacity for explicit targeting.

- *Health policy makers should be active in designing and strengthening national identification and targeting systems.* This will ensure that these systems develop in ways that can be used by health programs.

- *There is no "best practice" model capable of accommodating any country at any stage of development.* The best path to cover people is one that corresponds to the socioeconomic fundamentals of the country, invests in creating the institutions and capacities to manage an increasingly complex health system, and recognizes the need for frequent adaptation.

- *The quality of UHC programs' implementation often improves as they mature.* Learning is an essential ingredient for all those involved in transitioning to UHC, and requires investments in "UHC skills," which will, ultimately, pay off.

- *The road to UHC often uses stepping stones.* While some reforms create path-dependence, others do not, and the latter can play a useful transitional role. Some of the institutions analyzed in this book have such a role, allowing governments to initiate a transition to UHC using a bottom-up approach. Some such stepping stones are the autonomous programs targeting only the poor, as evidence from several countries shows they are a temporary step and can evolve in different directions. Policy makers and researchers should acknowledge that, because the road to UHC is long, some of the early choices may be suboptimal for the final configuration of the health system, but are still appropriate for a system in transition.

Expanding Benefits—Chapter 3

In expanding health care benefits through UHC programs, policy makers face a methodological difficulty of defining "universal coverage" for these benefits, as there is no clear finish line but rather a seemingly limitless list of possible additions. They must also consider many factors when deciding how to expand the benefits, including epidemiological and demographic conditions, the desire to balance objectives such as health outcomes and financial protection, and political economy considerations.

Key Trends

Most UHC programs are moving beyond services related to the Millennium Development Goals (MDGs) to provide inpatient or specialist outpatient care, but chronic disease management is still often weak, even as the associated disease burden rises. A few countries, however, are focusing on strengthening delivery of primary health care and health care services related to the MDGs.

While most countries articulate their own priorities in defining the benefit package, priority setting remains weak: half the programs use no formal prioritization criteria and many of them have no clear system for decision making. Also, changes to the benefit package are rarely accompanied by an assessment of its impact on costs to providers or to financiers.

Most countries are moving to a more explicit definition of benefit entitlements, usually through a "positive list," although some countries also use a "negative list." How the lists are defined varies, and may include health conditions, clinical procedures, and covered drugs. Still, only a few countries use standardized coding systems, making it harder to enforce and monitor policies or compare their outcomes.

Despite the increasing focus on explicit benefit packages, many countries show a gap between the package promised and the package actually available, particularly for the poor and those in rural areas, often mediated through implicit rationing.

The purchase of services is also changing, as new payment systems are introduced to improve the incentives facing providers in ways consistent with the challenges they face. UHC programs have modernized and innovated payment systems, such as performance-based top-ups for public facilities and closed-ended bundled payments for private facilities, so as to better align incentives with policy priorities like improving productivity, raising quality, or containing costs.

Policy Implications

- *A focus on priority setting using more systematic and institutionalized processes that consider evidence and stakeholder views is vital because resources will always fall short of the huge range of potential health care services.* These decisions for prioritizing benefit packages often require initial decisions on institutional structure, processes, and criteria. The criteria may include the country's disease burden, as well as scientific cost-effectiveness studies and health technology assessments.

• *Noncommunicable diseases (NCDs) seem to be the widest gap in service coverage, and need attention given their overwhelming share of the disease burden.* As in most countries globally, NCDs are the predominant causes of morbidity and mortality in the 24 countries in the Universal Health Coverage Studies Series (UNICO), but weak coverage makes them a key focus area for the future.

• *Delivering the promised coverage requires planning and effort.* Consideration of service availability and readiness, and preventing factors that curtail effective coverage, are as vital as the expansion design itself.

• *Strengthening programs' management capacity, particularly in contracting providers and purchasing strategically and effectively, will be vital.* UNICO countries have progressively developed the stewardship function of the government and its willingness to augment its capacity by engaging the private sector, using novel payment mechanisms, and starting to finance outputs rather than inputs. All of this means that program management is increasingly complex and needs upgraded capacity for contracting and purchasing.

Managing Money—Chapter 4

A major question for all UHC programs is how to pay for expansion in coverage, as well as the efficiency, equity, and effectiveness with which resources are raised, pooled, allocated, and used.

Key Trends

The median UHC program expenditure per beneficiary across UNICO countries in 2011 was US$39, about 1.4 percent of GDP per capita and 0.4 percent of GDP. The relatively low costs are because UHC program expenditures do not cover the full cost of providing care, as separate supply-side public expenditure channels have continued to cofinance public provision in most UNICO countries.

Government financing in expanding coverage for the poor is crucial: about 70 percent of revenues across all programs came from general government revenues, and coverage for the poor was noncontributory in all

24 UNICO countries. Perhaps surprisingly, half the countries have ear-marking in various forms to cofinance coverage expansion. With the partial exception of China, voluntary prepayments from the nonpoor informal sector were not a prominent source for expanding coverage, and despite the new UHC programs, out-of-pocket expenditure (OOPE) at the point of service by households remains a prominent source of overall health system financing in most UNICO countries.

Most UHC programs were not part of national, single-payer risk pools. In over two-thirds of the UNICO countries, risk pooling was fragmented with UHC programs coexisting with other parallel pools, with some operating nationally and others subnationally. In theory, UHC programs providing comprehensive coverage and embedded in single-program UHC initiatives provide several potential advantages for reducing fragmentation, promoting solidarity, and enabling cross-subsidization. In practice, other approaches have achieved these results: several countries have expanded coverage without following a single risk-pool model, including Colombia, Mexico, and Thailand; others—such as Chile with its Explicit Health Guarantees (AUGE) law that a decade ago reformed how the country runs its UHC program, Fonasa, and private insurers—have attempted to harmonize benefits without necessarily pooling financing; or Colombia, Jamaica, and Tunisia, which have explicitly cross-subsidized financing across risk pools without merging them. Also, several countries that *have* merged various subpopulations financed by different sources of revenue within the same institution are providing different benefit packages and allocating different per capita expenditures to each subpopulation, including Indonesia and Vietnam.

About half the UHC programs reported requiring some cost sharing by beneficiaries at point of service and, in most cases, these copayments were retained by facilities. Cost sharing is seen in about a third of inpatient programs, in about half of outpatient specialized programs, and in most drug and diagnostic-services programs. In most countries, however, cost sharing has been largely eliminated for basic services, including the cost-effective prevention and treatment of most communicable diseases and child services. A slower trend is also seen toward eliminating cost sharing for maternal services.

A wide range of resource-allocation modalities are seen across UNICO countries. In some, risk- and equity-based adjustments were prominent in intergovernmental fiscal transfers. Others used matching and results-based allocations to enhance the resource base and the effectiveness of UHC program financing. Some evidence of ring fencing of allocations across levels of care is also evident, although more systematic information is needed.

Policy Implications

- *Containing fiscal sustainability risks.* Given the reliance on government sources for financing pro-poor expansion, there should be a greater focus on assessing the overall macro-fiscal context of health financing. Some countries that have expanded coverage to the nonpoor informal sector have financed this expansion fully with general taxes. Detailed fiscal space analysis is needed, grounded in estimating accurate costs of providing coverage to those not covered and in assessing potential sources of additional government health spending to establish if other countries could follow that path.

- *Curbing rising fiscal sustainability risks from greater explicitness of benefit packages.* The move toward making benefit packages more explicit potentially exposes countries to other fiscal sustainability risks—from, for example, cost pressures, increased utilization rates, and adoption of expensive medicines and technology—especially as accountability mechanisms mature in currently lagging countries. Some UNICO countries have mitigated such risks by explicitly limiting or circumscribing benefits (programs in Argentina and Nigeria covered only maternal and child health benefits, for instance). But these risks loom large for countries that have promised open-ended comprehensive entitlements that are, in effect, not universally made available to all beneficiaries, leading to implicit rationing that disproportionately affects the poor and vulnerable.

- *Ensuring complementarity of demand-side and supply-side financing.* The majority of UHC programs provide demand-side financing, but traditional supply-side financing for publicly run health facilities continues to cofinance health coverage across most UNICO countries. This implies that issues related to public financial management and incentive compatibility are key in determining whether UHC programs will be successful in the move to UHC. Clear policy stipulations are needed on flexibly using demand-side funds, combined with strong accountability mechanisms.

- *Enrolling the nonpoor informal sector.* Some UNICO countries such as Chile, Costa Rica, and Turkey have enrolled the nonpoor informal sector using a contributory modality. Further analysis is needed to better understand how this was managed, and to identify key lessons.

- *Assessing the costs and benefits of earmarking.* Several countries use different forms of earmarking to finance UHC expansion. A key question is whether earmarked resources are truly additional, or whether they are largely displacing regular government financing. A stronger evidence base is needed to help determine whether earmarking should be recommended as an option for generating additional revenues, and if so, whether some forms of earmarking are preferable to others.

- *Understanding the persistence of OOPE.* OOPE remains high in many UNICO countries, despite rising coverage. Here, too, more research is needed on the extent to which OOPE reflects inadequate financing for UHC and poor supply-side readiness. Issues of financial protection should be accorded greater priority.

- *Sensitizing policy to progressivity of financing sources and cross-subsidization.* The diversity of pooling and resource allocation across UNICO countries underscores the need for policy to be sensitive to issues of progressivity of financing sources and cognizant of the extent of cross-subsidization in pooled funds across UHC programs. Resource-allocation modalities must be designed to ensure that financing is channeled to where it is needed the most, and not to create barriers to effective risk pooling and cross-subsidization.

Improving Health Care Provision—Chapter 5

While more financial resources may be needed for UHC, alone they will not be enough to deliver high-quality health care services—the health system has to be run in a way that ensures affordable access to them. UHC programs are closing this "provision gap" by improving their supply of services to meet the health care needs of their populations and the demand created by coverage expansion.

Key Trends

Human resources for health loom large in supply issues. To address distribution concerns—especially ensuring that health workers are available in rural and remote areas—UNICO countries have adopted outreach services via mobile health units and community health workers (CHWs). Many UNICO countries have also used monetary and nonmonetary incentives to attract and retain health workers, and to improve their performance. A combination of output-based payment methods and expanded benefit packages has produced more incentives for physicians and health care providers to increase production and availability of some services. Some UHC programs also improve health worker productivity by offering nonmonetary incentives, such as better work conditions, conference and training support, or even opportunities for higher education. UNICO countries are also attempting to boost human resource effectiveness by investing in their capacity and skills.

Efforts to expand the stock of resources include engaging with private providers and incentivizing public providers. About half the programs make use of private providers. Many UHC programs are also trying to improve the performance of publicly run health facilities by granting them more financial autonomy and flexible cash management at primary, secondary, and tertiary levels. While not enough is known about the efficacy of these reforms, it is known that not all incentive systems get it right at the first attempt and need to be monitored, and reformed, as they evolve.

To improve accountability and patient safety, most UNICO countries are introducing processes such as accreditation and improved regulation. Many of these processes are still reported to be weak in design and operation, illustrated by the fact that only a few UHC programs could identify actions taken against health care providers who failed to comply with guidelines or were involved in malpractice.

Most UNICO countries' policy makers appreciate the need for integration across the health system to ensure that the population has access to an organized, optimally functioning network of health care providers, but also understand the complexity of the task. Many UNICO countries have therefore started with a focus on primary health care, which is not only an obvious choice for better health outcomes, but also an essential first step to an integrated system.

Policy Implications

- *Policy makers need to consider the capacity of health care provision and enhance it, as necessary, to attain their UHC objectives.* Financing is important, but a UHC program is only as good as the services it can buy, and if they are unavailable when and where needed, any effort toward UHC will be incomplete.

- *A raft of tools can enhance the engagement, capacity, performance, and utilization of human resources for health.* Investments in their greater effectiveness are at the heart of efforts to enhance supply, and include better performance measurement, monetary and nonmonetary incentives to reward performance, and improvements to capacity and skills. The private sector can be leveraged to augment service availability.

Choice of public and private providers can also be a tool for improved accountability.

- *Good monitoring and oversight are essential, as are the ability and agility to make mid-course corrections.* Incentives do not always achieve the initially intended effects and may need to be revised over time, and so should be monitored closely.

- *Mechanisms to ensure quality of services contribute to patient safety and accountability, and should be integral to UHC program design and not presented as an afterthought.* Accreditation may offer some benefits, but also important are good regulatory oversight and other mechanisms like standard treatment guidelines.

- *Gatekeeping and referral mechanisms are complex, and most countries struggle to get them right, but they should persevere.* Well-performing health systems require attention to design, implementation, and monitoring. A focus on primary care contributes to a more sustainable, accessible, and equitable health system, attaining better health outcomes at lower cost.

- *Operational knowledge needs to be strengthened.* Key areas for further research include measuring the efficiency and quality effects of providing autonomy to health facilities or managers on human resources performance; analyzing the improvement in effective coverage linked to improvements in supply; describing the functions and implementation of integrated services in health care networks, including community outreach and an assessment of why primary health care clinics are bypassed; assessing the effects of mobile health units and CHWs on health outcomes in remote and poor areas; and measuring the impact on the quality of care of institutional arrangements to accredit health care providers.

Strengthening Accountability—Chapter 6

UHC programs across the 24 countries do much more than add people, services, or money to an existing health system. They aim to fundamentally change the way that stakeholders interact, with the objective of strengthening accountability among policy makers, providers, and the population. Accountability matters, both at a large scale to ensure that UHC programs achieve their objectives and that resources are used effectively; and at a micro scale to ensure that individuals and institutions meet their responsibilities. Using a framework popularized by the

World Development Report 2004, the chapter analyzes each of the major elements of an accountable relationship—delegation, finance, performance, information, and enforcement.

Key Trends

The first step toward stronger accountability is delegation. The case studies indicate that UHC programs are increasingly using arm's-length relationships (such as a purchaser-provider split, engagement of private providers, or autonomy for public providers) and identifying more explicitly different parties' roles and responsibilities (including explicit benefit packages and greater clarity in intergovernmental fiscal relations in federal states).

On finance, establishing more arm's-length relationships has been complemented by efforts to link the additional financing provided by the UHC programs to specific results, commonly seen in a partial shift toward output-based financing. Some countries do this at micro level, providing incentives for quality, productivity, or cost control through provider payments to hospitals, clinics, managers, or frontline workers. Others clarify fiscal relations by, for example, linking transfers to subnational governments to performance indicators. Outside service provision, financial incentives are often used to encourage agencies or jurisdictions to enroll priority populations.

Accountability also requires robust information. Nearly every UNICO case study cites heavy data collection efforts, and a few countries have signaled the importance of data reporting by directly incentivizing information provision. However, while some areas such as financial and technical audits are growing, there is minimal use of data for strengthening accountability or general monitoring and evaluation. Perhaps the biggest shortcoming is that fewer than half the UHC programs include regular reporting on health outcomes, financial protection, or equity—some of it attributable to lack of skilled staff in health care management and health economics, though other factors may also be at play, including political economy.

A final channel is empowering citizens. The case studies identified a wide variety of interventions to achieve greater client voice or power, typically involving measures providing greater access to information and to grievance-redress mechanisms. The former include access-to-information legislation, information campaigns, report cards that provide information on service performance to citizens, scorecards, and social audits; the latter are sometimes established in government agencies or independent organizations. But in some countries courts form the main redress mechanism, sometimes "judicializing" the right to health.

Policy Implications

- *The accountability measures related to delegation and financing were viewed favorably in the vast majority of case studies, and addressing their absence was a key reform cited in others.* This is especially true in middle-income countries where the capacity to implement these contractual arrangements is usually stronger. It is less clear that low-income countries should hasten to adopt the same measures, although there are some examples of success.

- *The experience of UHC programs in information and empowering citizens is mixed.* Many countries are either struggling in these areas (information), or have only made tentative measures (citizen/client power). In all countries, questions have yet to be answered on how to establish a culture of evidence-based policy making that draws on the new information—principally by applying well-developed monitoring and evaluation expertise—and how to empower citizens to hold politicians, policy makers, and providers to account for UHC implementation.

- *To strengthen accountability, greater effort is needed in information and empowerment.* In particular, more operational research is needed to help, for example, identify: who has established effective monitoring systems; how to implement information technology reforms; how to create stakeholder support for strong information flows; how and where to create analytical capacity for monitoring UHC programs; and how best to empower patients and citizens to hold providers and politicians accountable.

- *Very few UHC programs systematically measure program impact on key objectives such as better health outcomes and financial protection.* The reasons are not fully clear—whether it is a capacity constraint, political economy issue, or something else—but they warrant urgent attention, or the accountability agenda remains incomplete.

Conclusions—Chapter 7

The final chapter briefly discusses the key policy trends observed across the 24 countries, the key policy choices that countries make to chart their own path toward UHC, the stepping stones they often use along that path, and the new risks that must be addressed. As the first two have been detailed in the previous pages, here we focus on the latter two.

Stepping Stones

Countries often make choices that would be imperfect for a final configuration of a health system providing UHC but that make sense if understood as temporary. For example, programs targeting the poor and vulnerable are sometimes criticized as being incompatible with UHC, with critics arguing that universality should cover all populations. But many UNICO countries use these programs as a starting point and then expand them in different directions. The programs are thus useful in giving countries the chance to develop new skills in, for example, targeting, enrollment, output-based payments, and results-based budgeting.

Voluntary health insurance is also criticized for its inability to provide UHC but it, too, may serve as a valuable temporary solution providing some coverage as well as a smoother political transition, than inaction would, for the needs of the nonpoor informal sector at an early stage when the government's focus is on the poor and vulnerable.

Autonomous informal sector programs, operating separately from SHI, may also be transitory. They can rapidly expand, but generate a trade-off between equity and sustainability, which, in the long run, may require additional reforms.

Lastly, the coexistence of supply-side subsidies and demand-side payments may also be transitory. While the introduction of demand-side payments improves incentives, it is unclear how well the different sources of funds are being combined at local and facility levels—an area of future research.

This research plea in fact applies to several areas, for identifying which of these stepping stones allow countries to retain flexibility in designing future steps and which ones curtail it, creating "path dependence." The experience of the UNICO countries suggests that starting narrow and then broadening (from targeting the poor to broader population coverage) is relatively easy to do; starting broad and later narrowing (from having a wide benefit package and then curtailing items) is far harder.

New Risks

New approaches, new risks—in three areas. First, new programs are more complex and demand sophisticated technical and political capacities. Second, they involve explicit promises that generate expectations and create the risk of "broken promises" where actual outcomes fall short of expectations. Third, they may create new fiscal risks.

The UHC programs are not just about adding more resources to the system, but instead involve an attempt to introduce a new way of doing business that is more complex and requires new technical skills. The greater complexity is partly due to new activities not performed before (such as identifying and targeting subpopulations or explicitly prioritizing certain health care services) and partly due to new ways of implementing existing activities (such as operating with output-based payments or introducing financial audits). The new programs also compel greater political skills to manage the losers (winners don't complain), because they aim to change the way health systems are organized. These skills will be put to the test in, say, adopting explicit targeting or choosing the benefit-package expansion path from among those supported by powerful provider interest-groups.

Gaps between expectations and outcomes are prevalent in the UNICO programs, notably between the promised benefit package and the de facto benefits obtained by program beneficiaries, leading to widespread implicit rationing. The transition is also slow and incomplete on targeting, generating a gap between theoretical and real-life arrangements. Outcomes and expectations are rarely compared, even though large volumes of data are collected on multiple aspects of UHC programs. This wealth of data needs to be exploited, and the lack of monitoring and reporting (health and financial) rectified.

The move toward making benefit packages more explicit potentially exposes countries to fiscal sustainability risks, especially as some accountability mechanisms lag behind. Some UNICO countries have already attempted to mitigate these risks by explicitly limiting benefits or by limiting the promise to a certain subpopulation. Other countries have promised very generous entitlements and currently limit the fiscal impact by implicitly rationing access to the benefit package. As mechanisms of accountability become stronger in these countries, they may be forced to make their promises better fit their fiscal realities.

What We Know ... and What We Need to Know

Countries around the world are implementing UHC programs following a bottom-up approach that are new, massive, and transformational. These programs are expanding coverage in ways that are inclusive of the poor and are changing the way health systems operate, attempting to make these systems more efficient and equitable. Much of the available evidence suggests these programs may be reaching their objectives—but more operational research is needed to guide policy makers in their efforts to cover people, manage money, expand benefits, improve health care provision, and strengthen accountability. It is hoped that this book helps set the stage for a new generation of such research by identifying, at the minimum, the challenges that keep policy makers awake at night.

CHAPTER 1

Introduction

In health systems around the world, countries are going universal. The quest for universal health coverage (UHC) has gathered real momentum over the past decade or so, with countries on every continent now taking part. Looking out over the next 10 years, there is every reason to believe that this trend will continue.

This is very good news of course. A lack of universal coverage means that tens of millions of people around the world either do not get the health care services they need or they have to pay dearly for it, often falling into poverty as a result (WHO 2010). The heaviest burden falls typically on the poor and vulnerable. Thus achieving more rapid progress toward UHC is important for the broader global goals of ending extreme poverty and boosting shared prosperity. Making progress on this front is one of today's most important public policy imperatives.

The broader context for the push toward UHC includes steady income growth and the demographic and epidemiological transitions taking place around much of the globe. Emerging middle classes with a political voice, aging populations, and greater prevalence of chronic diseases mean that a growing number of people worldwide are now demanding better access to care and the potential for healthier lives that modern medicine can offer. A positive policy response to these forces can help achieve what has been called the "health financing transition," whereby health spending per capita grows and a larger share of total health expenditures is pooled (Savedoff et al. 2012). Politicians and policy makers are increasingly recognizing this demand, and are starting to act on it.

But there is much hard work to be done. The metaphor of a long journey seems most appropriate, as UHC cannot be achieved overnight, and although there is no unique path to UHC, a country's starting point matters a lot for the immediate road ahead. Much planning and preparation are required, but uncertainty along the way is to be expected, and course corrections made. And most important for this book, there is much to learn from fellow travelers.

Going Universal—A Focus on "How"

This book is about 24 countries that have embarked on that long journey. The main objective is to document and analyze their experiences based on a systematic data collection effort (see *Methodology—Countries, Programs, and Data*, this chapter) that sought to capture in great detail *how* they are doing so. Thus the book aims to extend, on number of countries covered and detail of information collected, the large number of case studies that have already enriched the global knowledge base on UHC (for instance, Tangcharoensathien et al. 2011; Knaul et al. 2012; Atun et al. 2013; Maeda et al. 2014; Marten et al. 2014; Saleh et al. 2014).

How to achieve UHC is admittedly not the first question likely to be asked by policy makers. What is UHC, and why their governments should make it a priority, are likely to be their initial queries (box 1.1). They have been addressed in greater detail elsewhere (WHO 2010; Jamison et al. 2013, for example).

What does it mean to ask "how" to achieve UHC? One possible response is to think about where the money will come from, which organization will manage these funds, and how the resources will be translated into health care services on the ground. These issues reflect the three core health financing functions of revenue generation, pooling, and purchasing. They embrace some of the classic debates about health system design, including sources of tax, third-party payers, public provision, and so on. These are essential considerations for any attempt to launch a UHC initiative, and have justly received quite a bit of attention in the recent UHC literature (Lagomarsino et al. 2012; McIntyre et al. 2013; Oxfam 2013; Rockefeller Foundation et al. 2013). They will also receive attention here.

Another common starting point for talking about how to chart a path toward UHC is to refer to the "UHC cube" popularized in the *World Health Report 2010* (WHO 2010). This depicts three dimensions of coverage—the population (who is covered?), services (which are covered?), and cost sharing (what proportion of costs are covered?). It conceptualizes the journey toward UHC as a task of making progress along each of these dimensions to help "fill" the cube (figure 1.1).

The UHC cube raises the real-world dilemma of which dimension to prioritize, given the inevitable trade-offs. Should more people get a smaller benefit package or fewer people a larger package? How can this

BOX 1.1
Before the "How"—"What?" and "Why?"

While this report focuses on "how" countries are aiming to achieve UHC, the "what?" and "why?" are also important for policy makers.

What is UHC?

UHC is about all people having access to the health care they need without suffering financial hardship. A few implications of this definition stand out.

First, taking the concept literally, it could be said that no country has yet achieved UHC, and that it is essentially an aspirational goal. But even if the destination is far off, for most countries the broad direction *toward* UHC is quite clear—for example, by addressing current shortcomings such as access barriers and high out-of-pocket expenditure (OOPE). Moreover, there is an ongoing effort to develop a substantive UHC monitoring framework that includes an overarching goal, targets, and indicators for service coverage and financial protection, including among the poor and vulnerable (World Bank and WHO 2014).

Second, this formulation should also make it clear that UHC is not just a matter of "counting people" who are (or not) part of a particular program—it is not binary. There are many dimensions, including the services available, their quality, and how much the patient must pay.

Third, UHC can be seen as a repackaging of the long-standing goals of all health systems, such as access, quality, equity, and ultimately better health and financial protection. In this sense, UHC may be seen as "new wine in an old bottle" (Wagstaff 2013), and on the substance of the ultimate goal, that may well be true. But as this report will show, the instruments that countries are using to achieve these goals are very much evolving.

Fourth, the emphasis on objectives should also free us from thinking that only one instrument (insurance, for example) is consistent with UHC. Instead, UHC can be achieved through a wide range of approaches.

Lastly, because in most countries the richest segment of the population is usually much closer to having full coverage than the poor, the task at hand can also be seen as narrowing current inequalities in health systems.

Why should countries pursue UHC?

There are several good answers. Perhaps the most common is to assert that health (and implicitly UHC) is a *basic human right*. This view is consistent with Article 25 of the Universal Declaration of Human Rights (1948). It is also enshrined in many national constitutions, with important implications for UHC programs.

Perhaps a more pragmatic approach is to argue that UHC reforms often make for *good politics*. As incomes grow and basic needs are met, one of the first demands made by emerging middle classes is for better access to health care. They represent an important electorate, and politicians have often seized on that to win their support by promoting UHC efforts. The launch of many UHC reforms can in fact be traced to important political events such as newly elected governments.

Finally, there are strong *economic reasons*. The health sector, and especially health insurance, is subject to pervasive market failures that justify government intervention. And rates of return to health spending are often very high (on average, if not always on the margin) because modern medicine at its best can make a huge difference to health, and people attach very high value to better chances of living a long, healthy life. As a result, UHC programs represent a potentially very high benefit-to-cost ratio for governments seeking value for money from their limited budgetary envelope (Jamison et al. 2013).

FIGURE 1.1
The UHC Cube

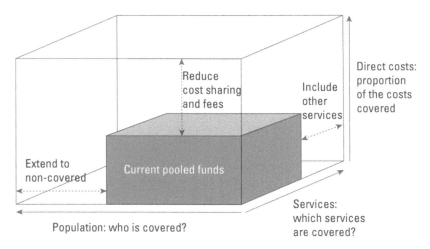

Direct costs:
proportion
of the costs
covered

Reduce
cost sharing
and fees

Include
other
services

Extend to
non-covered

Current pooled funds

Services:
which services
are covered?

Population: who is covered?

Source: WHO 2010.

balance be altered by the level of cost sharing to be required? This
approach of how to achieve UHC has also received attention in the literature. Most notably, the recent Lancet Global Commission 2035 analyzed
alternative "pathways to progressive universalism," and espoused support for two options (Jamison et al. 2013). The first would make coverage
available to the whole population but target the poor by prioritizing
health interventions for diseases that disproportionately affect that group.
The second would provide a larger package of interventions to the full
population but with some patient copayment, from which poor people
would be exempt. It also explicitly rejects pathways that propose heavy
reliance on private voluntary health insurance or "catastrophe-only"
health insurance plans.

But for policy makers who wish to learn about the nuts and bolts of
UHC implementation, answering the question of "how" must go beyond
a discussion of broad approaches. Instead, practical implementation
issues are the order of the day (Bennett, Ozawa, and Rao 2010). To continue the metaphor of a long journey, just as the decision to travel by air,
rail, or sea cannot fully define a long trip, so the pursuit of UHC cannot
be reduced to a choice among a few alternative macro models or pathways. Instead, any country's UHC model embraces dozens of elements
across a wide range of domains. It is only by fully unpacking these features that we can attain a more complete understanding of the choices
to be made, as well as guidance on implementation issues.

Some illustrative questions can help convey this. For example, is the
benefit package defined by service level or disease, or not defined at all?

Is a costing of the program needed? Are revenues earmarked? Do participating facilities have to be accredited? What, if any, new institutions should be created? If so, to whom are they accountable? How do people enroll, or should enrollment be required at all? Do beneficiaries get an ID card or not? What are the information reporting requirements? How will the public express their views? The list of questions could go on for many pages.

These more specific questions have arguably received inadequate attention thus far during policy discussions on UHC, which have instead focused on "macro issues" such as whether to adopt an insurance model or not. But most countries pursuing UHC reforms have already made these macro decisions, and so it is on these more specific components that they need greater guidance in charting a path. This book aims to shed some light on them by drawing extensively on global experiences.

Methodology—Countries, Programs, and Data

This book is based on systematic data collection among 26 UHC programs across 24 countries in the Universal Health Coverage Studies Series (UNICO) around the world (map 1.1). Before proceeding to the thematic chapters that constitute the core of this document, it is important to briefly explain how these countries were selected and what the data collection effort entailed. Some important caveats are also in order. Basic indicators on the countries are presented in appendix B.

The 24 countries were selected on the basis that over the past decade or so they have made substantial efforts to strengthen coverage of health care services from the "bottom up." That is, they have recently expanded coverage with a special focus on the poor and with the overarching objective of attaining UHC. Some 30 countries were identified that fit these criteria. Of these, an effort was made to collect data on as many programs as possible, resulting in a total of 26 programs from 24 countries across six regions. (In India, three UHC programs were included to reflect the diversity of bottom-up UHC expansion programs in that country). Through the book, we refer to the reforms implemented by these countries as "UHC programs." This is not intended to imply that these countries have achieved UHC, as that is a very long-term goal (see box 1.1). Rather, the term is used as shorthand to refer to programs that aim to make significant strides toward UHC with a focus on the poor and vulnerable.

A focus on the past decade or so implies overlooking a large part of the history of UHC worldwide. The first step toward UHC in the modern era was famously taken in Bismarck's Germany during the late 19th century. Over the course of the first half of the 20th century, most other

MAP 1.1
Countries in This Book's UNICO Studies

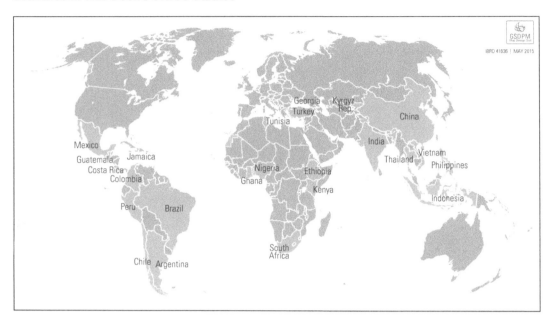

Source: UNICO studies.

industrialized countries followed suit. By the 1970s, arguably every rich country except the United States had achieved some approximation of UHC for its citizens. Among low- and middle-income countries, there were some early successes achieved 50 years ago, including in Eastern Europe, the Soviet Union, and elsewhere, such as Cuba, Malaysia, and Sri Lanka (though they all have unfinished agendas). Instead, our focus begins with those countries such as Brazil and Colombia, which initiated reforms in the 1990s. But it was only in the first years of the new millennium that the latest wave of UHC reforms really took off, beginning with the launch of Thailand's Universal Coverage Scheme (UCS) in 2001. Reforms aimed at UHC in the most populous middle-income countries such as China, India, and Indonesia are less than 10 years old.

The selection of countries based on a focus on the poor also entails missing part of the UHC picture. It is possible to make important advances in pursuing UHC without an explicit focus on the poor. Health systems with a population-wide orientation have sometimes achieved very equitable outcomes, but in many cases government health spending is largely captured by the better off (chapter 2). Still, the focus here on UHC programs working from the bottom up does imply a certain sample bias.

In brief, the programs do not constitute an exhaustive list of all UHC reforms around the world today, and so do not capture every country experience from which important trends can be identified and lessons drawn. Nevertheless, together they account for programs covering over one-third of the world's population, or some 2.5 billion people, and therefore offer an important data set from which to learn about UHC worldwide (map 1.1).

Table 1.1 lists the programs and basic coverage statistics. The programs vary widely on population coverage, ranging from less than 1 million to over 800 million, and from less than 5 percent to 100 percent of the country's population. The average coverage rate is 45 percent. These programs expanded rapidly between 2006 and 2011, adding nearly 1.5 billion people. Over half the programs have more than doubled their coverage rate over this short time.

The data collection tool for the UNICO studies comprised a common "Nuts & Bolts" questionnaire with nine modules and 329 quantitative and descriptive questions (appendix D). Its modules collected information on, among other areas, a country's health system, the history and institutional architecture of the selected program within each country, details of beneficiary targeting and enrollment, management of the benefit package, data on public financing of the program, cost containment, and the information environment. Decentralization of service delivery was the focus of a supplementary module. Most respondents were World Bank country teams engaged in project support and policy dialogue. Data collection activities were completed in 2012, with key coverage, financing, and other indicators referring to 2011. Based on the information compiled for the questionnaire, a series of country case studies were drafted in advance of an author workshop held in 2012.

The unit of analysis is the UHC program, not entire health systems, although much contextual information about the latter was collected. This unit was chosen so as to focus on what is new or changing, since this is where reforms have been concentrated. Overall health systems change only slowly, as it is just not possible to replace one system wholesale with another, but there is a risk in this approach that we lose sight of the system due to an exclusive focus on the program, thereby potentially failing to capture the impact (positive or negative) of a targeted UHC program on the entirety of a country's population (Kutzin 2013). UHC, after all, is about everyone. But inevitably there exists some trade-off between scope and depth of analysis, and the advantage of this approach is that it allows for a much deeper understanding of how nascent UHC programs are functioning and evolving. In addition, as will be shown, the UHC programs are often serving to leverage broader reform of health systems, effectively blurring the distinction between the two.

Appendix C shows the results of a systematic review of the literature on impact evaluation. This exercise identified over 6,500 studies

TABLE 1.1
Population Covered by the 26 UHC Programs, 2006 and 2011

Country	UHC program	UHC program coverage (millions)		UHC program coverage (% of total population)	
		2006	2011	2006	2011
Argentina	Maternal-Child Health Insurance Program (Plan Nacer, MCHIP)	0.4	1.7	1.0	4.3
Brazil	Family Health Strategy (Programa Saúde da Família, FHS)	86	102	45	51
Chile	National Health Fund (Fondo Nacional de Salud, FONASA)	12	13.2	68	78.0
China	New Rural Cooperative Medical Scheme (NRCMS)	410	832	32	64
Colombia	Subsidized Regime (SR)	14.3	22.3	32.5	47.4
Costa Rica	Social Security of Costa Rica (Caja Costarricence de Seguridad Social, CCSS)	3.9	4.3	88.6	91.5
Ethiopia	Health Extension Program (HEP)	8.9	60.9	11.4	68.1
Georgia	Medical Insurance Program (MIP)	0.3	0.9	5.7	20.0
Ghana	National Health Insurance Scheme (NHIS)	2.5	8.2	11.4	32.8
Guatemala	Expansion of Coverage Program (Programa de Extensión de Cobertura, PEC)	3.8	4.4	29.2	29.3
India	National Rural Health Mission (NRHM)	0	840	0	70
	Andhra Pradesh Rajiv Aarogyasri (RA)[a]	0	70	0	85
	Rashtriya Swasthya Bima Yojna (RSBY)	0	70	0	6
Indonesia	Jamkesmas	60	76.4	26	32.0
Jamaica	National Health Fund (NHF)	0.3	0.5	11.0	19.0
Kenya	Health Sector Services Fund (HSSF)	0.0	20	0.0	48
Kyrgyz Republic	State-Guaranteed Benefit Package (SGBP)	4.0	4.2	76.0	76.0
Mexico	Popular Health Insurance (Seguro Popular, PHI)	15.7	51.8	14.3	43.2
Nigeria	Ondo State National Health Insurance Scheme (NHIS-MDG-MCH)[a]	0	0.1	0	4.0
Peru	Comprehensive Health Insurance (Seguro Integral de Salud, SIS)	10.4	12.7	37.1	42.3
Philippines	National Health Insurance Program (NHIP)	68.5	78.4	79.0	82.5
South Africa	Antiretroviral Treatment Program (ATP)	0.3	1.5	0.6	2.7
Thailand	Universal Coverage Scheme (UCS)	47.5	47.7	72.0	71.2
Tunisia	Free Medical Assistance for Poor (FMAP)	2.4	3.0	24.1	27.0
Turkey	Green Card (Yesil Kart)	8.3	9.1	12.0	12.4
Vietnam	Social Health Insurance (SHI)	23.4	55.4	28.2	63.0
Total/average		781.9	2,390.8	27.1	45.0

Sources: UHC program coverage data from UNICO questionnaires, supplemented by government documents. Coverage rates are World Bank's calculation based on World Development Indicators (2014) and US Census Bureau.
a. The programs in India/Andhra Pradesh and Nigeria/Ondo State are both state-level programs, thus coverage is estimated for state populations.

attempting to evaluate UHC program impact on access to services, on financial protection, and on health outcomes. Despite the success of individual studies to stir debate leading to program adjustments in the countries studied, in the aggregate this literature is not very useful as a *guide* for policy makers facing the next generation of UHC reform challenges because in the aggregate the results are inconclusive and do not tell us *why* some programs have an impact—and others do not.

The main limitation comes from the effort to compare the impact of UHC programs without controlling for the many differences that exist across programs. In this book we show each UHC program involves several components, that each component requires choices and that the quality of implementation of the individual components matters. The programs are different in how they cover people (targeting just the poor and vulnerable or also covering the nonpoor informal sector?); how they expand benefits (including inpatient care or only outpatient care?; does it contract providers using fee for service or other payment systems?); how the provision of services is improved (integrated networks, private-provider participation, some public-provider autonomy?). If a program does not have an impact, the existing methodology is incapable of identifying which component of the program is "not working." A new generation of operational research needs to unbundle the programs into their key components and examine if each component "works." A huge challenge no doubt, but one that needs to be overcome by researchers interested in finding answers to the operational questions facing policy makers.

While this book does not attempt to establish the impact of the policies reviewed on key outcome indicators, it hopes to help policy makers and researchers by providing a more granular understanding of the individual policies or components that together constitute an overall reform program. For policy makers the book seeks to identify areas of policy consensus, areas requiring choice and the risks involved in the different choices; awareness of these trends from around the world can serve as a mirror to their own system and provide new ideas of what can be tried. For researchers, it hopes to provide a more granular understanding of the challenges and policies requiring evaluation.

Attacking Inequality—The Common Starting Point for Diverse Paths to UHC

The starting point for bottom-up UHC programs is, in a single word, *inequality*. The poor get much less from their health systems than the rich. Unequal health systems are unequal in many different ways.

The poor are often in a different subsystem (for example, managed by the MoH [Ministry of Health] instead of a social insurance agency) with less funding per person. They may not have access to the same providers as the rich, and get substandard care as a result. Or those providers are reimbursed at a lower level for the poor and thus cut corners or turn them away. The poor often cannot pay for even small costs for care if they are not covered, such as drugs or medical supplies that are out of stock. When there is implicit rationing (see chapter 3, *Defining Benefits—Toward Explicit Benefit Packages*), the rich can often use their connections (or money) to jump the queue. The poor may live in rural areas where good care is hard to find. Or public spending may be heavily concentrated on a tertiary hospital in the capital city. The poor may also belong to historically disadvantaged groups, such as ethnic minorities, who face discrimination when they seek care. Inequality has many causes.

The extent of inequality resulting from these features has become amply clear in recent years. As discussed in chapter 2, empirical evidence over the past decade or so has drawn attention to inequalities in utilization of essential services between rich and poor: public expenditure studies reveal a pro-rich bias of government health spending, and measures of financial protection point to the common risk of catastrophic and impoverishing health spending by the poor and vulnerable (Filmer 2003; Wagstaff et al. 2014). For policy makers faced with this evidence, the imperative is to mount an attack on inequality (Yazbeck 2009).

While inequality is the common starting point for the bottom-up UHC programs studied in this book, countries have chosen very different pathways. Their choices reflect many considerations, from different levels of development to specific calculations of what is possible for them. Differences across programs may suggest that any analysis amounts to comparing apples and oranges, but in fact it is this diversity that offers rich insights into the options for implementing UHC programs.

The case studies reveal that countries are adopting one of two broad approaches to bottom-up UHC. The first, referred to here as a "supply-side program (SSP)," channels investments to expand the capacity of service provision through more funding for inputs (for example, human resources) and reforms such as greater flexibility in staff recruitment, financial autonomy for public clinics, strong organizational protocols, and explicit performance indicators. Eight such programs are among the 26 (table 1.2). They are "bottom up" because they focus on the services typically used by the poor—in six out of eight countries the focus is on primary care, often with an emphasis on rural areas.

TABLE 1.2
Typology of UNICO Programs

Supply or demand side	Target population mix	Autonomous or embedded in SHI	Name of model	UHC programs (based on 2011 status)
Supply-side	Open to all populations but focuses on services typically used by poor	Not applicable	Supply-side program (SSP)	Brazil (FHS) Ethiopia (HEP) Guatemala (PEC) India (NRHM) Jamaica (NHF) Kenya (HSSF) Nigeria (NMM) South Africa (ATP)
Demand-side	The poor and vulnerable	Autonomous from SHI	Poor and vulnerable program (PVP)	Georgia (MIP) India (RA) India (RSBY) Indonesia (Jamkesmas) Peru (SIS) Tunisia (FMAP) Turkey (Green Card)
	All informal sector population (including the poor and vulnerable)	Autonomous from SHI	Informal sector program (ISP)	Argentina (Plan Nacer) China (NRCMS) Colombia (Subsidized Regime) Mexico (Seguro Popular) Thailand (UCS)
	Poor and vulnerable embedded with formal sector population in SHI	Embedded in SHI	Poor and vulnerable program embedded in SHI (SHI+)	Ghana (NHIS) Kyrgyz Republic (SGBP) Philippines (NHIP) Vietnam (SHI)
	All informal sector populations (including the poor and vulnerable) embedded with formal sector population in SHI	Embedded in SHI	Informal sector program embedded in SHI (SHI++)	Chile (Fonasa) Costa Rica (CCSS)

The second broad approach encompasses "demand-side programs" that attach resources to a specifically identified poor and vulnerable population and the services they use. These programs identify and enroll their target population and strategically purchase health care services on their behalf via output-based pay. The countries following this approach can be further divided into four groups according to who is covered and to whether the program is autonomous or embedded in the formal sector program (often a social health insurance agency): poor and vulnerable program (PVP), informal sector program (ISP), poor and vulnerable program embedded in SHI (SHI+), and informal sector program embedded in SHI (SHI++). These categories are discussed in greater detail in chapter 2.

Irrespective of which approach is taken, all UHC programs seek to address both a "financing gap" (lower spending per capita on the poor) by spending additional resources in a pro-poor way and a "provision gap" (underperformance of service delivery for the poor) by seeking to change incentives in a host of ways. Thus most UHC practitioners (policy makers and program operators) appear to have converged around a view that the road to UHC will require not just more money but also a laser-like focus on changing the rules of the game around how health system resources are spent.

A Guide to the Book

The objectives of this book are to document and interpret key trends in the implementation of UHC based on a systematic data collection effort across 24 countries to help guide work by UHC implementers around the world. The main intended readers are policy makers engaged in UHC (in UNICO countries and elsewhere), especially practitioners in ministries of health and finance. It also aims to reach an audience in broader policy circles engaged in UHC issues in these countries and globally, including think-tanks, academia, civil society, and international agencies.

Chapters 2, 3, and 4 correspond roughly to the three dimensions of the "UHC cube": people, benefits, and money. Chapter 5, on improving health care provision, builds on chapter 3 (benefits) to look at service delivery. Chapter 6, on accountability, looks at some means by which stated objectives within each of the other topics are met and ensured. In slightly more detail:

- *Chapter 2—Covering People* addresses how to extend UHC to a larger population. While the ultimate goal of universal (100 percent) coverage is clear, few countries with incomplete coverage can achieve this quickly, and thus some priorities must be set and mechanisms put in place to enroll some, but not all, people. The focus is on the poor and vulnerable, and the nonpoor informal sector.

- *Chapter 3—Expanding Benefits* discusses choices related to adding more services to coverage programs. If only some services can be afforded, it is not obvious how to select them, how to define the benefits to be offered, and how to contract with providers to deliver care.

- *Chapter 4—Managing Money* addresses the classic issues of health financing, including revenue generation, pooling, and purchasing (broadly defined). These are core questions for any UHC program and a key concern for ministries of finance. Intergovernmental fiscal relations are also discussed.

- *Chapter 5—Improving Health Care Provision* shifts the focus from people, benefits, and funding, on paper, to the actual delivery of health care services, on the ground. UHC can be an empty promise if infrastructure, human resources, pharmaceuticals, and high-quality integrated care are not easily accessed by the population needing them. This chapter looks at what countries are doing to avoid this.

- *Chapter 6—Strengthening Accountability* examines the wide range of interventions aimed at fundamentally changing the relationships between key stakeholders, with the objective of making them more accountable to each other. Accountability is critical to ensure program success overall and that all individuals and institutions fulfill their responsibilities.

- *Chapter 7—Conclusions* summarizes the key chapter messages and draws out implications for the UHC agenda. It identifies key policy choices as countries pursue UHC and their implications. It highlights the common use of "stepping stones" or transitional arrangements to UHC—that is, policies that are quite clearly imperfect for a final configuration of a health system but that make more sense if understood as temporary solutions along a lengthy reform trajectory. Lastly, it identifies some new risks for UHC programs, including managing increased complexity of the health system, the often wide gap between promised reforms and actual outcomes, and challenges of fiscal sustainability.

Finally are the appendixes. Appendix A lists the 26 UNICO studies and authors. Appendix B presents some basic indicators on the UNICO countries. Appendix C provides a literature review of impact evaluations of UHC programs, where the few studies undertaken have tended to focus on program impact overall, rather than the effectiveness of individual components. Appendix D reproduces the Nuts & Bolts questionnaire used to collect information across the studies.

References

Atun, R., S. Aydin, S. Chakraborty, S. Sümer, et al. 2013. "Universal Health Coverage in Turkey: Enhancement of Equity." *The Lancet* 382 (9886): 65–99.

Bennett, S., S. Ozawa, and K. D. Rao. 2010. "Which Path to Universal Health Coverage? Perspectives on the World Health Report 2010." *PLoS Med* 7 (11): e1001001.

Filmer, D. 2003. "The Incidence of Public Expenditures on Health and Education." Background note for World Development Report 2004: Making Services Work for Poor People, World Bank, Washington, DC.

Jamison, D., L. H. Summers, G. Alleyne, K. J Arrow, et al. 2013. "Global Health 2035: A World Converging within a Generation." *The Lancet* 382 (9908): 1898–955.

Knaul, F., E. González-Pier, O. Gómez-Dantés, D. García-Junco, et al. 2012. "The Quest for Universal Health Coverage: Achieving Social Protection for All in Mexico." *The Lancet* 380 (9849): 1259–79.

Kutzin, Joe. 2013. "Health Financing for Universal Coverage and Health System Performance: Concepts and Implications for Policy." *Bulletin of the World Health Organization* 91: 602–11.

Lagomarsino, G., A. Garabrant, A. Adyas, R. Muga, and N. Otoo. 2012. "Moving towards Universal Health Coverage: Health Insurance Reforms in Nine Developing Countries in Africa and Asia." *The Lancet* 380 (9845): 933–43.

Maeda, A., E. Araujo, C. Cashin, J. Harris, N. Ikegami, and M. Reich. 2014. *Universal Health Coverage for Inclusive and Sustainable Development: A Synthesis of 11 Country Case Studies.* Washington, DC: World Bank.

Marten, R., D. McIntyre, C. Travassos, S. Shishkin, W. Longde, S. Reddy, and J. Vega. 2014. "An Assessment of Progress towards Universal Health Coverage in Brazil, Russia, India, China, and South Africa (BRICS)." *The Lancet* 384 (9960): 2164–71.

McIntyre, D., M. K. Ranson, B. K. Aulakh, and A. Honda. 2013. "Promoting Universal Financial Protection: Evidence from Seven Low- and Middle-Income Countries on Factors Facilitating or Hindering Progress." *Health Research Policy and Systems* 11: 36. doi:10.1186/1478-4505-11-36.

Oxfam. 2013. "Universal Health Coverage: Why Health Insurance Schemes Are Leaving the Poor Behind." Oxfam Briefing Paper 176, Oxfam GB, Oxford, United Kingdom.

Rockefeller Foundation, Save the Children, UNICEF, and World Health Organization. 2013. "Universal Health Coverage: A Commitment to Close the Gap." Save the Children, London. http://www.rockefellerfoundation.org/uploads/files/57e8a407-b2fc-4a68-95db-b6da680d8b1f.pdf.

Saleh, S., M. S. Alameddine, N. M. Natafgi, A. Mataria, et al. 2014. "The Path towards Universal Health Coverage in the Arab Uprising Countries Tunisia, Egypt, Libya, and Yemen." *The Lancet* 383 (9914): 368–81.

Savedoff, W., R. Bitrán, D. de Ferranti, V. Y. Fan, et al. 2012. *Transitions in Health Financing and Policies for Universal Health Coverage: Final Report of the Transitions in Health Financing Project.* Washington, DC: Results for Development Institute.

Tangcharoensathien, V., W. Patcharanarumol, P. Ir, S. M. Aljunid, et al. 2011. "Health Financing Reforms in Southeast Asia: Challenges in Achieving Universal Coverage." *The Lancet* 377 (9768): 863–73.

Wagstaff, A. 2013. "Universal Health Coverage: Old Wine in a New Bottle? If So, Is That So Bad?" *Let's Talk Development* (blog), February 12. http://blogs.worldbank.org/developmenttalk/universal-health-coverage-old-wine-in-a-new-bottle-if-so-is-that-so-bad.

Wagstaff, A., M. Bilger, L. R. Buisman, and C. Bredenkamp. 2014. "Who Benefits from Government Health Spending and Why? A Global Assessment." Policy Research Working Paper 7044, World Bank, Washington, DC.

WHO (World Health Organization). 2010. *The World Health Report—Health Systems Financing: The Path to Universal Coverage.* Geneva: WHO.

World Bank and WHO. 2014. "Monitoring Progress towards Universal Health Coverage at Country and Global Levels: Framework, Measures and Targets." http://apps.who.int/iris/bitstream/10665/112824/1/WHO_HIS_HIA_14.1_eng.pdf?ua=1.

Yazbeck, A. 2009. *Attacking Inequality in the Health Sector: A Synthesis of Evidence and Tools.* Washington, DC: World Bank.

CHAPTER 2

Covering People—The Bottom-Up Approach

This chapter emphasizes two developing-country features that add granularity to a discussion of population coverage: the population is segmented into subpopulations that relate to the health system in different ways[1]; and universal health coverage (UHC) programs are not about covering populations that previously had zero coverage—all countries in the study already offer something to everyone. Public health care services, usually provided by the Ministry of Health (MoH), are available in all the 24 Universal Health Coverage Studies Series (UNICO) countries. The problem is that too often what is available for everyone is not very good, such that the poor are left behind.

In the early 2000s, evidence came through that publicly financed health care services in most developing countries greatly favored higher-income groups. A study of spending patterns in 21 such countries found that in 15 of them public spending favored the highest-income groups, while only four provided a larger subsidy to the poor (Filmer 2003; World Bank 2004). Another study on 56 developing countries found that health programs designed to advance the millennium development goals (MDGs) were expanding coverage, but were doing so following a "trickle-down" approach evidenced by coverage rates that were about two-thirds higher for the richest 20 percent than for the poorest 20 percent (Gwatkin, Wagstaff, and Yazbeck 2005). This evidence led to an appreciation that, left to their natural inertia, efforts to expand health coverage in unequal societies naturally drift toward a trickle-down approach (figure 2.1).

Countries seeking a more progressive path to UHC have developed strategies that prioritize the expansion of access to health care services and to financial protection for lower-income populations. We refer to these strategies as a "bottom-up approach" to expanding health coverage. At its core this approach draws on the recognition that different strategies

FIGURE 2.1
Trickle-Down and Bottom-Up Expansion of Health Care

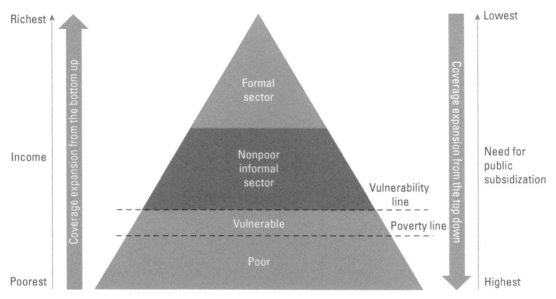

are required to attend to the needs of each subpopulation (or segment). The bottom-up approach became possible because developing countries had acquired new capacities, allowing them to give preferential treatment to segments that had traditionally been left behind in the expansion of health coverage. This chapter describes how these new capacities are used to expand health coverage in more progressive ways—"from the bottom up."

Segmented Populations, Fragmented Health Systems

The population of the 24 UNICO countries has three large segments (figure 2.2).

The *formal sector* is composed of salaried workers and their families. These families tend to be in the upper half of the income distribution. A key characteristic is that they are relatively easy to tax via payroll taxes. At the turn of the millennium, 18 of the 24 countries operated a social health insurance program (SHI) based on salaried workers' compulsory payroll taxes; these taxes were earmarked to provide health coverage to these workers and their families.

The *nonpoor informal sector* is composed of nonsalaried workers and their families with incomes above the vulnerability line. The income of this segment is harder to tax than salaried workers' income, and at the

FIGURE 2.2
Health Systems in UNICO Countries before the Introduction of UHC Programs

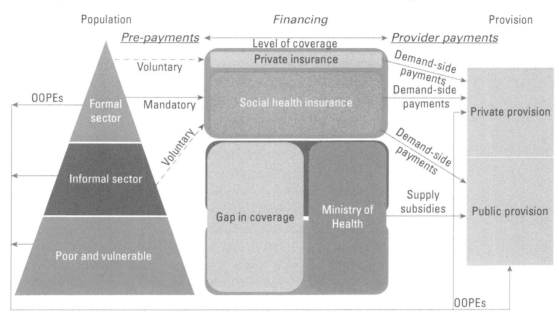

turn of the millennium few UNICO countries had developed compulsory contribution systems for this subpopulation. As a result, people in this segment would normally pay for services out of pocket, using private providers or higher-end services offered by public providers.

The *poor* cannot afford to pay for health care and risk falling deeper into poverty if they have to pay for health care costs. The *vulnerable* are above the poverty line but health care expenditures can easily drag them below it. At the turn of the millennium all UNICO countries covered these two groups with services subsidized by the MoH (or equivalent).

Coexistence of an MoH with an SHI was almost the norm across most UNICO countries in 2011 (the year for which the UNICO study collected the comparative data)—18 of the 24 countries had this configuration (and see table 1.2). In addition, two countries had previously had this configuration but had merged the two systems into one in recent decades (Brazil and Costa Rica). Of the remaining four countries, one created a national health insurance program in 2013 (Georgia), and two are considering creating a national health insurance program (Ethiopia and South Africa), which would coexist with MoH services.

Figure 2.2 illustrates relations between the three subpopulations, the health financing system, and public and private providers in countries with an SHI and an MoH, before UHC programs were introduced.[2] Private insurance covered a small group of the higher-income population financed through voluntary payments. In about half of the UNICO countries the SHI also provided coverage to a small group of informal sector families, who paid voluntary contributions to enroll. The MoH, financed by general taxes, covered the rest of the population, including the non-poor informal sector, and the poor and vulnerable.

MoH coverage as measured by per capita spending was typically narrower than that provided by the SHI or private insurance. The higher per capita spending by an SHI usually implied that the formal sector population had access to more benefits (such as breast cancer treatment) and was subject to either no or lower copayments for those benefits than the rest of the population served by the MoH (for example, no copayment for deliveries). The narrower MoH coverage left a "financing gap in coverage" for the nonpoor informal sector and the poor and vulnerable.

Private and public providers were financed by out-of-pocket expenditure (OOPE) by users at the point of service and by prepayments channeled through the MoH, SHI, and private insurers. The SHI and the MoH financed the supply of services using different procedures. The MoH financed such supply by public providers by paying for inputs used for the provision of services (health workers, pharmaceuticals, etc.). These payments subsidized the direct cost to the users and are referred to as "supply subsidies." By contrast, SHI typically paid providers for "outputs" (services and goods) provided to SHI enrollees; these payments are "demand-side payments."[3]

Fragmentation of the health system occurred not only in health financing, but was also common in service provision. In most of the 24 UNICO countries the better off and the poor rarely used the same health care facilities, especially at primary and secondary levels of care, which were commonly characterized by unresponsive services that imposed high transaction costs on users in the form of long waiting times, the need for repeated visits, and often discourteous treatment (table 2.3 below). This generated a form of "implicit targeting," as the better off self-selected away from these services.

Integrated use of facilities by the better off and the poor was only common for tertiary care, although at that level the better off had greater access to high-cost technology and to specialists than the poor. Typically, the MoH had some higher-end services for which fees were charged in urban hospitals, and lower-end services in rural and peri-urban areas which had eliminated or reduced fees, especially for interventions related to communicable diseases and to maternal and child care (chapter 3). Public providers frequently offered more attractive services for paying users than for the poor.

These two features (segmented populations and fragmented health systems) were among those that UHC sought to overcome. After all, achieving UHC is primarily about covering all people. It is individuals and households who suffer the consequences of poor access to health care services and a high financial burden when they seek care. Reflecting this, the most common metrics of UHC involve counting people—for example, how many do or do not have coverage, or how many face catastrophic or impoverishing OOPE. How to cover more people is therefore a good place to begin a discussion of implementing UHC.

Identifying and Targeting the Poor—And Getting Better at It

Identifying the poor across the vast landscape of a country is not easy, although the UNICO studies suggest that the 24 countries are getting better at it. The past two decades have seen tremendous gains in these countries' capacity to identify the poor, as they move to more rigorous and transparent methods. These change over time as the countries learn to balance the costs and benefits of the new techniques, for targeting involves heavy costs in multiple areas. The literature (these costs were first discussed by Besley and Kanbur 1990) recognizes three types of associated costs:

- *Administrative and informational costs.* Accurately distinguishing between who is and who is not poor and vulnerable entails costs, including the cost of the means used to identify individuals and households and the administrative costs of gathering information about their socioeconomic status.

- *Incentive costs.* These arise when eligibility criteria induce households or other participants in UHC programs to change their behavior in an attempt to become beneficiaries. For example, a program that makes informal sector workers eligible for the same benefits as formal sector workers without having to pay for these benefits may encourage growth of the informal sector, with consequent costs to the economy.

- *Political costs.* These costs arise in the form of political opposition to the program.[4]

A first wave of instruments and institutions was developed during the 1990s that allowed governments and donors to identify *regions* with large numbers of poor people. This information was initially used to prioritize these regions for investment in small-scale infrastructure. To better target these investments, countries developed information systems, producing "poverty maps" of regions with high concentrations of poor people, which were often combined with maps identifying geographic gaps in social infrastructure. These poverty maps helped prioritize investment for poor areas, triggering further institutional innovation in public investment procedures as many countries developed simpler procedures for small investments in civil works that involved grassroots organizations in planning and supervising those investments (Jack 2001).

At this point it is useful to distinguish between the eight supply-side and 18 demand-side programs. The supply-side programs aim to improve the quality, accessibility, and attractiveness of services within a specific jurisdiction or for people with a certain health condition. These programs often target regions and services used by the poor (box 2.1), rather than individuals or households (as is done by demand-side programs).

More recently, many middle-income countries and an increasing number of low-income countries—including many of the countries implementing UNICO's 18 demand-side programs—have developed increasingly sophisticated techniques to identify poor *households* or *individuals* within a region (box 2.2).

Many UNICO countries are now using a combination of box 2.1's methods to identify, target, and enroll individuals or households eligible to benefit from social assistance programs, in a marked improvement from earlier, spatial systems. The institutions that implement these techniques and manage the lists may be labeled "targeting registries" (TRs).[5] In 2011, 17 of the 24 UNICO countries had set up a TR. That year, eight of the 26 UHC programs were using such a "TR" system to establish eligibility for UHC programs and five others were using one as a complementary instrument to ensure that people identified as poor by the TR obtained health coverage.

TRs are essential for demand-side programs and UNICO countries are increasingly using them. In 2012, Indonesia and Turkey switched from community-based targeting by local governments to more rigorous methods of identifying the poor and vulnerable through a central TR. In Ghana, the UHC program had been inaugurated with a mandate to cover the indigent. Initially it had only been able to use demographic targeting because it had no TR, but in 2013 the program adopted this approach.

How TRs are used is changing over time. Colombia and Mexico have powerful TRs that have served as global models for other countries setting up theirs. These two countries, plus Thailand, originally targeted all public subsidies to the poor using a TR and charging the nonpoor to participate in the UHC programs. These three countries have abandoned the attempt to raise contributions from the nonpoor informal sector and instead are extending full subsidies to all their informal populations (see later this chapter). They continue to use the TR but only to design outreach activities that motivate and inform the poor about the benefits of the UHC program, and no longer use them to identify beneficiaries.

BOX 2.1
Targeting Populations with Supply-Side Programs

The Brazil FHS is a program characterized as universal and its charter is to cover the entire population. Yet despite its universalist mandate, this supply-side program was prioritizing the poor fairly well in 2008 (figure B2.1.1). Its coverage of the poorest quintile was very high and coverage diminished as income climbed. Macinko (2011) explained that three mechanisms were behind this.

FIGURE B2.1.1
Distribution of UHC Program Coverage by Family Income Quintile, Brazil, 2008

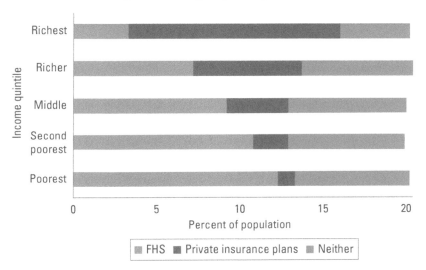

First was geographic targeting. After 15 years, the program covered over half the national population. Over time it had been rolled out in a way that prioritized the poorest municipalities and by the time of the study it covered almost all the poorer municipalities but was present in only half the richer ones. The second mechanism was self-selection—a large proportion of the population in the top quintile is covered by private insurance and opts out of the FHS. This opting out is incentivized through tax exemptions for private health insurance. Third, in some municipalities, promoting the outreach and enrollment of all households receiving the conditional cash transfer in FHS further incentivizes coverage of the poor.

Source: Macinko 2011.

The experience of Chile and Costa Rica is different. They continue to use TRs based on proxy means tests as a first step to identify the poor and vulnerable, but the UHC programs, working with tax agencies, now use means testing to estimate the income of beneficiaries in their efforts to increase revenue collection from nonpoor populations.

BOX 2.2
Targeting Methods

Community-based targeting uses a group of community members or leaders to decide who in the community should benefit from, for example, a social assistance program. School officials or the parent–teacher association may determine entry to a school-linked program; a group of village elders may determine who receives grain for drought relief, etc. The advantage of such targeting is that it relies on local information on individual circumstances and permits local definitions of need and welfare. Conversely, it may lower the cohesion of local communities if anyone is perceived to benefit unfairly.

Demographic targeting is based on age and on the rationale that individuals may be particularly vulnerable in childhood and old age. It is administratively simple and carries the appeal of universality, and is thus often politically popular. The limitation is that age may be only weakly correlated with poverty.

Proxy means tests generate a score for applicant households based on fairly easy to observe household characteristics, such as location and quality of the household's dwelling, its ownership of durable goods, its demographic structure, and the education and occupations of its adult members. The indicators to calculate this score and their weights are derived from statistical analysis of data from detailed household surveys of a sort too costly to be carried out for all applicants to large programs. Eligibility is determined by comparing the household's score against a predetermined cutoff. The advantage of proxy means tests is that they require less information than true means testing, although administering them requires a large body of trained staff and moderate to high levels of data and processing capacity. The indicators are often not made public to avoid "gaming" by applicants, and the results may seem mysterious or arbitrary to some households and communities.

Means-test targeting is usually regarded as the gold standard of targeting. It seeks to collect nearly complete information on households' income or wealth (or both), and verifies the information collected against independent sources. Where suitable databases exist and agencies cooperate, information may be verified by cross-linking the registries of say, the welfare agency, property registrars, tax authorities, social security agencies, and the like. When this is impossible, households may be asked to submit copies of records of transactions, such as pay stubs, utility bills, or tax payments.

Means testing is most appropriate where declared income is verifiable, where some form of self-selection limits applications by nontarget groups, where administrative capacity is high, and where benefit levels are high enough to justify the costs of administering a means test. Some of the UNICO countries started with rudimentary systems and refined them gradually.

These targeting methods are applied using two different approaches. In a survey sweep approach all households in an area are interviewed and registered in a nearly exhaustive system, offering a better chance of reaching the poorest, who are likely to be less informed than others. In an application approach households have to come to a local welfare office or designated site to apply for benefits.

Source: Grosh et al. 2008.

The decision to adopt a TR needs to take into account the political costs of adoption, which—even when the TRs already exist—can be high. Before 2009, the Philippines used community-based targeting applied by local governments, which identified several million people as poor and led to their enrollment in health insurance financed by the central government. In 2009, the central government imposed a more rigorous methodology managed by a TR—the National Household Targeting System. The new system revealed that only 800,000 of the beneficiaries qualified as poor and were thus eligible for subsidies, yet it also found that many households that were poor had not been enrolled in the subsidized health insurance program. These findings generated tension between the central government, which promoted the National Household Targeting System, and local governments, which were faced with the political cost of dropping existing beneficiaries. Eventually an accommodation was found as most local governments opted for paying the premium for the population that was not financed by the central government (local governments can pay for the near poor and define the vulnerability line according to local conditions), and the SHI matched this effort by expanding the benefits included in the package, making enrollment more attractive.

Identifying beneficiaries includes creating credible identification (ID) systems for individual beneficiaries linked to information systems that tie UHC programs to providers. This is an area of rapid change and high variability across countries. In 2011, most UHC programs issued their own ID cards, ranging from simple cards with no photograph in Vietnam, through cards requiring annual stickers proving membership renewal in Ghana, to smart cards incorporating biometrics in India's RSBY. A few of the UHC programs used national ID cards (Thailand). The cards sometimes used a system of numbering issued by the UHC program (Argentina, Brazil, Mexico, and Indonesia, for example); in other countries there was already a big effort to use unified national ID numbering systems (China and Colombia). In many countries the system of identification worked reasonably well for the household head, but was a challenge for dependents (the Kyrgyz Republic or the Philippines), where poor households often did not have birth certificates).

Identifying beneficiaries at enrollment is a different process from identifying them at point of service. Information links between the UHC program and providers are complex: in some countries printed lists were issued to a provider assumed to be in charge of the households in its catchment area, but, for example, the area had not always had not been demarcated, patients often used a different local provider from the one with access to the list, and referral systems were not always defined. After several years of operating with these problems, the Philippines in 2013 launched an enrollment drive to link beneficiaries to primary providers, incentivized through a capitation arrangement. At the higher end of sophistication, providers operating in India's RSBY network were required to invest in smart card readers, biometric readers, and other associated hardware and software that allowed for instantaneous paperless connections and registration of transactions.

After identifying the poor and vulnerable, demand-side programs must then enroll them.

Enrolling People—Two Phases, Two Paths

Enrollment is a key element in UHC programs—23 of the 26 programs require it. In demand-side programs its main benefits are to target fiscal subsidies to selected populations and, in programs with a contributory approach for the nonpoor, to charge contributions. Beyond these functions, the case studies show that enrollment systems can develop into an instrument of management and behavior change in demand- and supply-side programs (box 2.3).

The country case studies suggest that most countries using the bottom-up approach follow a sequence when creating demand-side programs. During an initial phase, most establish programs targeted exclusively to the poor. Years later, this is followed by a second phase when the programs expand to cover the rest of the informal sector. During the initial phase, countries usually have voluntary health insurance programs for the nonpoor informal sector, allowing families to voluntarily enroll in a system that requires payment (but uptake of these voluntary programs is usually extremely low, as seen below).

All countries following the bottom-up approach acknowledge that health coverage for the poor must be fully subsidized by general taxes (chapter 4). When countries enter the second phase and attempt to massively cover the nonpoor informal sector, they have taken two different paths: some chose a contributory path, requiring nonpoor informal families to contribute toward their health coverage; others a noncontributory path, extending the use of tax subsidies provided to the poor to the rest of the informal sector.

In both phases, some countries embedded the program within an existing SHI program and other countries set up an autonomous agency to run the program (sometimes linked to the MoH) (table 2.1; and see table 1.2). This mode of operation is especially important during the second phase, as it is often associated with the two paths used to finance participation of the nonpoor informal sector.

Countries that embed the UHC program within the SHI follow the contributory path when enrolling nonpoor participants (regardless of

BOX 2.3
Benefits of Enrollment

In UHC programs the enrollment function has gone beyond targeting subsidies and receiving contributions, to offering other benefits.

Providing incentives to enroll. It is not enough to make the poor "eligible" for enrollment. It is often necessary to reach out to eligible households to explain the health advantages of enrollment, the way the process operates, and what it costs. Sixteen of the UHC programs provide financial incentives to the enrollment agency to encourage such outreach. India's RSBY pays insurers a premium per each family below the poverty line enrolled in the program; Argentina's Plan Nacer pays provincial governments for each pregnant mother enrolled in the official beneficiary lists; Brazil's FHS pays municipalities per "health team implemented" (that is, a certain number of families registered). Different programs assign the responsibility for enrolling beneficiaries to different agencies or use a combination of agencies; among UNICO programs, 11 used the UHC program, 11 local governments, and 7 health care providers. In addition to the incentives provided to the enrollment agency, there may also be financial incentives for users, often conditional cash transfers (CCTs) requiring, say, immunization, nutritional counseling, or growth monitoring.

Empowering users. Enrollment establishes a formal contract between the UHC program and the enrollee. A membership card can serve as a symbol that empowers users to demand their right to health care. Programs often make the benefit package explicit and provide complaint mechanisms, making it possible for users to know what their rights are and how to demand them. Examples include Peru's SIS, Mexico's Seguro Popular, and India's RSBY.

Establishing separate accounts for each beneficiary. Once the accounts are created—a high bar— information systems can allow each account to be monitored. Some of the UHC programs use these accounts to track transactions and spending by beneficiary, sometimes limiting their liabilities. For instance, Georgia's MIP, China's NRCMS, and India's RSBY provide reimbursements up to a certain speci- fied amount per year per beneficiary. Yet the UNICO study found that most programs have not developed the capacity to track expenditures and use of services of individual households. The questionnaire (appendix D) requested basic data on the use of outpatient and inpatient services and on average amounts reimbursed per beneficiary, but only very few programs could provide this information, and most that did used household surveys as a source, instead of administrative data.

Meeting health program population targets. Primary health care (PHC) programs have targets related to the population of a catchment area; programs treating HIV/AIDS or noncommunicable diseases (NCDs) target individuals.

Source: UNICO studies.

TABLE 2.1

The 18 Demand-Side UNICO Programs by Target Subpopulation and Links to SHI, 2011

Target population/ relation with SHI	Embedded in SHI	Autonomous agency
Poor and vulnerable	**Cell A** Ghana (NHIS) Kyrgyz (SGBP) Philippines (NHIP) Vietnam (SHI)	**Cell B** Georgia (MIP) India (RA) India (RSBY) Indonesia (Jamkesmas) Peru (SIS) Tunisia (FMAP) Turkey (Green Card)
Nonpoor informal sector	**Cell C** Chile (Fonasa) Costa Rica (CCSS)	**Cell D** Argentina (Plan Nacer) China (NRCMS) Colombia (Subsidized Regime) Mexico (Seguro Popular) Thailand (UCS)

Source: UNICO studies.
Note: The programs in Turkey and Indonesia switched from being autonomous to being embedded in SHI after 2011; see text for details.

whether they are from the formal or informal sectors). Countries that set up autonomous agencies cover only the poor during the first phase; once they enter the second phase they usually extend the tax subsidies to the nonpoor informal sector (table 2.1).

Most demand-side UHC programs of countries taking the bottom-up approach initially develop as programs for poor and vulnerable populations, targeting public subsidies to them only. In 2011, 11 of the 18 demand-side programs were at this stage. Seven of these were operated by autonomous agencies (cell B in table 2.1), while four countries had embedded these programs within their SHI systems (cell A).

The programs that today cover the entire informal sector further illustrate the pattern of starting with the poor, but also suggest that this phase is transitional. Programs in Argentina, Colombia, Mexico, and Thailand, which in 2011 were open to all the informal sector population (cell D), had evolved from programs initially targeting the poor (cell B): Thailand's UCS originated from an earlier program targeted to the poor (the Medical Welfare System); Mexico's Seguro Popular and Colombia's Subsidized Regime were inaugurated with a design that included a full subsidy only for the poor and required the nonpoor to pay contributions; Argentina's Plan Nacer—a program to reduce maternal and child mortality among the uninsured—initially focused exclusively on the poorest provinces. Finally, Turkey's Green Card program became part of that country's social security system (which also includes coverage for the nonpoor informal sector) in 2012.

During the initial phase, the institutional affiliation of the targeted programs tends to be a matter of controversy and often shifts during the life of a program (moving between the second and third column in table 2.1), reflecting political pressures and policy choices behind the contributory or noncontributory path to cover the nonpoor informal sector. In 2011, Peru's SIS and Turkey's Green Card were linked to the MoH, within government there was a big debate about shifting the affiliation to the social security agency (in 2012 as seen, Turkey's Green Card became part of that country's SHI). In 2011, Indonesia's Jamkesmas was autonomous from SHI, with links to the MoH (cell B in table 2.1), but subject to pressures to transfer it to the SHI, which took place in 2013. Administration of the RSBY and Georgia's MIP was outsourced to private health insurers in 2011, and both programs have now been transferred to the MoH.

Some analysts are concerned that the creation of programs targeting the poor create fragmentation and may lock countries permanently in a certain path, but the UNICO study finds little evidence to support these concerns. Programs targeting the poor are created within health systems that are already fragmented, and these programs tend to be transitional, often forming stepping stones toward more equitable, integrated systems that cover various population groups (box 2.4).

Five UNICO countries are using programs to cover the informal sector that are autonomous from the SHI agency (Argentina, China, Colombia, Mexico, and Thailand—see table 2.1, cell D). These programs depend mainly on general tax revenues (only China makes an effort to charge a fee for affiliation, but even there this fee covers less than one-fourth of the cost of the program), and attach great importance to high enrollment.

These programs' targeting systems aim to limit leakage of fiscal subsidies to the subpopulation covered by SHI. They endeavor to compare the database of beneficiaries of the UHC program covering the informal sector with the database of the SHI program covering the formal sector. This comparison is designed to allow the UHC program to limit reimbursements to their own beneficiaries and to permit health care providers to demand payment from the SHI for services rendered to their beneficiaries. But as the two databases were not designed for this, efforts to make this comparison are onerous, especially in countries that do not have a robust unique identifier.

Four of these five programs (all but China) targeted the poor and vulnerable before they expanded coverage to the rest of the informal sector

BOX 2.4
Does the Bottom-Up Approach Create Poor Services for the Poor?

A concern is that targeting efforts to the poor will create services that cater exclusively for them and that those services will lack the political clout that middle-class users bring to the services they use. But the UNICO programs did not target this way.

The supply-side programs are not creating services from scratch but modify existing services, aiming to improve quality and accessibility of public providers. Services for the poor existed before the UHC programs were introduced and segregation was already a significant feature in these systems (table B2.4.1). Brazil's FHS, Ethiopia's HEP, and India's NRHM greatly expanded in rural areas the availability and number of health care workers, drugs, and diagnostic capacity. Guatemala's PEC expanded the choice of providers to include nongovernmental organizations, and piloted a program to reimburse transport costs incurred by poor mothers travelling to well-equipped maternal hospitals that served a broader population. South Africa's ATP made treatment for HIV/AIDS available nationwide.

TABLE B2.4.1
Segregating the Better Off and the Poor in Health Care Provision
Percent

	Do the better off and the poor use the same facilities?	When they do use the same facilities, do they use the same:	
		High-cost technology	**Quality of the room within a hospital**[a]
Primary care (outpatient)	36	61	41
Secondary care	40	35	41
Tertiary care	73	22	69

Source: UNICO studies.
Note: Percent represents the share of UNICO countries for which a "yes" answer was obtained.
a. Indonesia has VIP, first-, second-, and third-class rooms.

In contrast, the demand-side programs seek to eliminate the financial barriers that made it hard for the poor to use more and better services than previously. In the Philippines' NHIP, the central government pays the insurance premium for the poor to enroll. In the Kyrgyz Republic's SGBP, which requires a copayment for certain services at the point of use, the poor (and other social groups) are exempted from it, and facilities are instructed to retain 10 percent of the revenue obtained from copayments to help finance this exemption. In rural China, where the NRCMS requires beneficiaries to pay three elements—a fee, deductibles, and copayments—the Medical Assistance Program covers these expenses for the poor.

(figure 2.3, second and third blocks). Colombia and Mexico were pioneers in developing systems to identify the poor and continue to use their TRs to ensure that the poor are included as program beneficiaries. Once the decision to expand the subsidies to the nonpoor informal populations was taken, some of these countries expanded coverage very rapidly. Studies describing the process in Thailand show that the speed of expansion was possible because of the work done during the previous decades in building up the networks of health care providers in the right locations. Also, the new policy took advantage of the skills developed in previous decades in enrollment and the strategic purchasing of interventions (Towse, Mills, and Tangcharoensathien 2004).

These five autonomous programs face a difficult trade-off between equity (in terms of the benefit package provided compared with the benefits provided by the SHI) and financial sustainability. The pressures to equalize benefits of the autonomous program with those of the SHI are enormous. Argentina, Colombia, Mexico, and Thailand have a history of social and community mobilization around the right to health. In Mexico and in Thailand there have been years of intense debate about equalizing the benefits of the autonomous informal sector program with those of the SHI. In Mexico, several successive governments have implemented a policy of annual expansion of the benefits of the Seguro Popular, and the reduction of the gap between the two programs is used as a measure of

FIGURE 2.3
Noncontributory Path to UHC

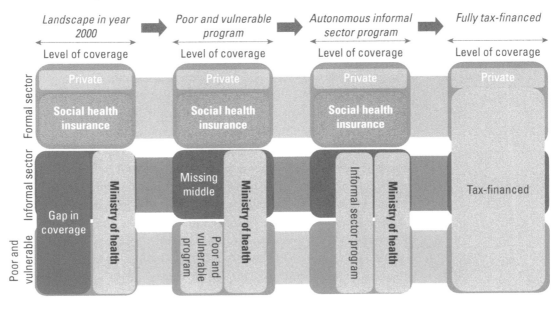

Note: The second and third blocks correspond to cells B and D, respectively, in table 2.1.

progress toward UHC (Knaul et al. 2012). A similar debate flared in Colombia for over a decade, leading to a Constitutional Court decision in 2008 ordering the government to equalize the benefit package of the Subsidized Regime with that of the Contributory Regime—this decision precipitated major health sector and tax reforms. In 2011, Argentina's Plan Nacer covered only reproductive, maternal, neonatal, and child conditions; the benefits and the eligible subpopulations were expanded sharply in 2013, but remain narrower than those offered by the SHI system. (The relatively narrow coverage of the autonomous programs is illustrated in the third block of figure 2.3.)

The problem of sustainability arises from the incentives these programs create for job-seekers. Levy (2008) first suggested that these programs may delay the formalization of the economy because workers will prefer informal to formal employment to avoid payroll deductions if the benefits in both sectors are similar. Several studies conducted in recent years for Colombia, Mexico, and Thailand provide some support to this hypothesis: for Colombia, Camacho, Conover, and Hoyos (2013) found an increase in informal employment associated with the introduction of the Subsidized Regime of 2–4 percentage points; for Mexico, Aterido, Hallward-Driemeier, and Pages (2011) using panel data found that the Seguro Popular may have increased labor informality by 0.4–0.7 percentage points; for Thailand, Wagstaff and Manachotphong (2012) found that Thailand's UCS appears to have reduced formal-sector employment, at least among some categories of the labor force.[6,7]

Bitran reviewed programs used to enroll informal sector populations in 13 countries and concluded that a narrower benefit package may be inherent to the autonomous informal sector programs: "… offering a uniform benefit package for all, just like offering free enrollment for the poor and the nonpoor informal alike, may result in such large perverse behaviors that the aim of achieving UHC may become infeasible" (Bitran 2014, i).

Resolving this trade-off between equity and sustainability may require ambitious health system reforms. The tension originates from the existence of two programs with opposing philosophies on the use of contributions to finance health coverage for the nonpoor. The SHI requires that the nonpoor should contribute to health care, regardless of whether they work in the formal or informal sector. The autonomous informal sector program operates separately from the SHI and rarely requires contributions from nonpoor informal sector groups (China is the only exception among the UNICO programs). Countries with both systems require some of the nonpoor to pay for health coverage but allow others with similar incomes to be exempt. In the long run, solving this equity/sustainability trade-off may involve a tax reform that eliminates reliance on payroll taxes to finance health care for the formal sector (see figure 2.3, last block).

While undertaking a reform of this nature represents a steep challenge for countries struggling to increase tax revenues, precedents exist. An example from a developing country is Brazil, which made its health system fully general-tax financed in the years following its constitutional reform of 1989. In the 1970s and 1980s, some Organisation for Economic Co-operation and Development (OECD) countries also reformed their health systems, moving from SHI and replacing it with general tax financing, such as Denmark (1973), Italy (1978), Portugal (1979), Greece (1983), and Spain (1986) (Saltman, Busse, and Figueras 2004, cited by Bitran 2014). Among the UNICO countries, this type of reform has been under consideration in recent years in Colombia, Mexico, and Thailand.

Six UNICO countries had embedded their UHC programs in their SHI systems by 2011 (Ghana, the Kyrgyz Republic, the Philippines, Vietnam, Chile and Costa Rica—see table 2.1, first column); more recently, Turkey and Indonesia have also transitioned to this model. Countries that have *recently* begun implementation of these programs (all except Chile, Costa Rica, and Turkey) cover the formal sector (financed by payroll contributions) and the poor (based on tax-financed transfers from the treasury), but make enrollment voluntary for the nonpoor informal sector and cover only a fraction of this sector. During this phase (second block of figure 2.4), the programs do not have the capacity to enforce mandatory contributions from informal sector workers; countries often offer partial subsidies for voluntary health insurance for nonpoor informal sector participants, but this attracts only a small fraction of the sector.

In 2011, the younger UNICO programs embedded in SHI (Ghana NHIS, the Kyrgyz Republic SGBP, the Philippines NHIP, and Vietnam SHI) had enrolled only a small part of the nonpoor informal sector, and participation of informal workers was based on voluntary contributions. During this phase (the second block in figure 2.4), countries often experiment with new measures that would allow them to enforce mandatory contributions from parts of the informal sector. For example, in 2013 the Philippines approved regulations that require municipalities to make renewal of municipal licenses for moto-taxi drivers and for market-stand permits conditional upon proof of health insurance. In 2010 the Peruvian Congress considered (but rejected) making such proof a condition for commercial loans to informal firms. These revenue collection efforts involve coordination among agencies, often across levels of government, requiring UHC programs to work with national and municipal tax collection agencies, property registries, and pension systems. Achieving collaboration across these agencies is challenging and requires time, as most of them have little incentive to share

FIGURE 2.4
Contributory Path to Covering the Informal Sector

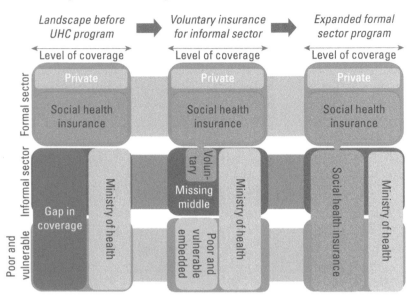

Note: The second and third blocks correspond to cells A and C, respectively, in table 2.1.

such access. A crucial first step is the creation and implementation of a common numeric identifier.

As the capacity to enforce contributions from the informal sector grows, these programs tend to incorporate progressively larger segments of the informal sector (last block of figure 2.4). In the more mature programs of the study (Chile's Fonasa, Costa Rica's CCSS, and Turkey's SHI after 2012) participation of the poor and the informal sector is de facto mandatory: the poor are fully subsidized by general taxes and the non-poor informal sector is subjected to a careful review of income using a raft of mechanisms. Turkey, for example, developed a sophisticated system to determine contributions for the self-employed. Contributions are proportional to a scoring system that depends in part on the household's taxable or estimated income, on the value and size of the property it occupies, and on the size and age of the car it owns.

But while some countries in the contributory path have enrolled many informal workers and collect contributions from them, revenue collection from such workers remains a challenge. For example, in Chile an enquiry in 2010 found that roughly 400,000 individuals were illegally enrolled as indigents. Voluntary health insurance may indeed be helpful during the initial phase of the bottom-up approach to UHC, but it is not a path to UHC (box 2.5).

BOX 2.5
Voluntary Insurance

Voluntary health insurance is not a path to UHC. Most high-income countries using health insurance to cover their population have recognized this by making such insurance mandatory and by providing subsidies for low-income subpopulations (most recently, the United States implemented this mandate as part of the Affordable Care Act).

Two recent reviews for developing countries confirm that voluntary health insurance is rarely successful in enrolling a large part of the informal sector population. Bitran (2014) reviewed 13 developing countries, many of which had a special window to enroll informal sector families in SHI programs, and found that these voluntary programs led to very low informal sector enrollment, even if many countries used partial subsidies to incentivize enrollment.

Bitran finds that even if enrollment is low in relation to the total population, these windows can be costly as they invite adverse selection: enrollees tend to comprise a large number of members with a high health risk and with large families. Thus when these schemes are managed by SHI agencies, they often become a financial drain on it and are often discontinued or discouraged. Argentina, Indonesia, and Peru have a long stop-and-go history in which these programs are created during periods of fiscal affluence, then discontinued or discouraged in fiscal downturns—and once more "rebooted" when fiscal and political conditions are propitious.

The effectiveness of subsidies and other incentives to enrollment have been recently studied using randomized control trials. Wagstaff (2014) documents experiments carried out in the Philippines and in Vietnam, where treatment groups were offered a subsidy (50 percent and 25 percent, respectively), information packages (including enrollment forms), and help in completing and submitting the paperwork. In neither country did the treatment groups come anywhere close to 100 percent enrollment: in the Philippines, the intervention increased enrollment from 10 percent to just 15 percent around a year later; in Vietnam the most effective intervention raised enrollment from 6 percent to just 7 percent a year later. A slightly more successful experiment was documented in Nicaragua by Thornton et al. (2010), but even there enrollment reached only 20 percent.

Insurance programs in rural China and in Rwanda have achieved high enrollment (the only two documented to do so worldwide). While formally they were "voluntary," they use enrollment procedures that involve local authorities whose performance is judged by their success enrolling the population in their jurisdictions. Their success in enrollment is associated with political forms of organization that are not easily replicable elsewhere.

The large number of studies and conferences devoted to providing proof that voluntary insurance is not a path to universal coverage may suggest that analysts assume that policy makers are unaware of the limitations of this approach. This does not seem consistent with the sophisticated understanding and huge appetite for knowledge displayed by these same policy makers in other topics, however. A more plausible hypothesis might be that policy makers understand that it is not a path to universal coverage, but serves as a palliative for certain problems and as a political escape valve that is useful while countries become capable of covering the nonpoor informal sector, either by mandating contributions or by financing their coverage with general tax revenues.

Using Fundamentals and Investing in Learning

Countries need to assess realistically their options for implementing UHC programs based on their socioeconomic fundamentals, and should invest in learning the capacities needed for implementation. The challenges of extending health coverage to nonpoor informal sector workers and their dependents are huge: the informal sector may account for 80–90 percent of the population in low-income countries and around 40–50 percent in middle-income countries (ILO 2013), and many of them are nonpoor (figure 2.5). It is also vital to raise revenues from this population as they are undertaxed compared with the formal sector; tax revenues forgone from the informal economy have been estimated to be as high as a third of all potential tax revenue in developing countries (Cobham 2005, cited by Bitran 2014).

The biggest challenge is for the poorest countries, as they generally have larger informal sectors, higher poverty ratios, and lower government revenues to finance health care. With few exceptions, UNICO countries that ranked above the median on share of informal sector in total employment also have poverty ratios above the median and per capita gross domestic products (GDPs) below it (figure 2.5). The figure serves as a vivid reminder that when we refer to developing countries as a whole, we are combining countries such as Turkey, Argentina, Costa Rica, and Brazil—with informality rates of around 50 percent and poverty ratios in the single digits—with countries such as India, Kenya, or Ethiopia—with informality rates of around 90 percent and poverty ratios of over 65 percent. Per capita GDP in international dollars in the first group is multiple times higher than in the second group.

While comparable household survey data are not available for all UNICO countries, the methodology used to produce the case studies required an assessment of countries' success in covering the informal sector. Based on that assessment, only eight countries have achieved significant coverage of their informal sector. The highest rates of coverage of the informal sector were achieved by (in alphabetical order): Argentina, Brazil, Chile, China, Costa Rica, Mexico, Thailand, and Turkey. All these countries have informal sectors as a share of total employment smaller than the median for the UNICO countries in figure 2.5. In other words, even in a group of countries chosen because they have made significant efforts to expand coverage of their populations during the past decade, there is a clear relationship between the socioeconomic fundamentals and progress in those efforts.

FIGURE 2.5

Share of Informal Employment and of Poor Populations, Selected UNICO Countries

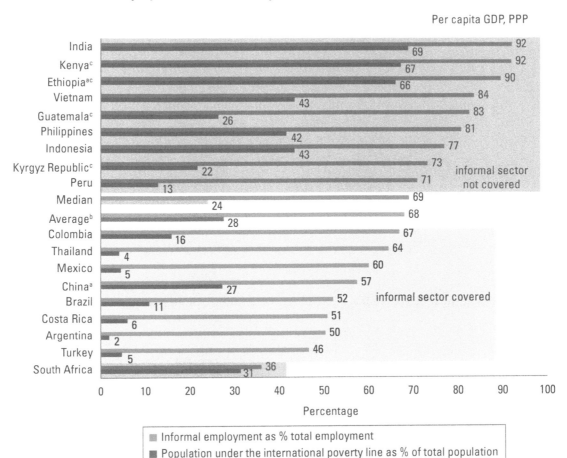

Source: Key Indicators of the Labor Market (ILO 2013) for informal employment as percentage of nonagricultural employment, and for the relative size of agricultural sector. World Development Indicators (World Bank 2014) for persons in poverty as a percentage of total population. World Bank's calculation for the relative size of informal employment in total assuming all agricultural employment is informal. All data are for the latest possible years, between 2008 and 2010. World Economic Outlook (IMF 2014) for GDP per capita (PPP) information for year 2013.

a. Data for informal employment as % of nonagricultural employment are from subnational surveys: conducted in six cities in China and urban areas in Ethiopia.

b. Unweighted average

c. Data for Ethiopia, Guatemala, Kenya, and Kyrgyz Republic refer to "persons employed in the informal sector" instead of "persons in informal employment."

Does the Choice of Model Matter?—Achieving Two Intermediate Objectives

The long-term objective of UNICO countries is UHC. In the shorter run countries attempt to achieve two intermediate objectives that are often used as indicators of how well programs cover people: enrollment of the poor and vulnerable and of the nonpoor informal sector; and prioritizing the poor in the distribution of public subsidies (limiting "filtration" to nontargeted groups).

How well countries achieve these intermediate objectives can be illustrated by household survey data, used for eight UNICO countries. Of the eight, five had programs targeting the poor and three had programs covering the entire informal sector. Three had programs embedded in SHI and five had autonomous programs (table 2.2).

There is a significant variation in the degree of success with enrolling the poor and vulnerable: some of the countries have enrolled most of the

TABLE 2.2
Model and Maturity of Selected Programs by the Time of Household Survey

Country	Name of UHC program	Model in year of household survey		Year of UHC program creation	Year of household survey	Maturity[a]
		A or SHI	PVP or IS			
Thailand	Universal Coverage Scheme (UCS)	A	IS	2002	2009	34[a]
Turkey	Green Card	SHI	IS	1992	2011	19
Colombia	Subsidized Regime (SR)	A	IS	1993	2011	18
Peru	Comprehensive Health Insurance (SIS)	A	PVP	2002	2011	9
Indonesia	Jamkesmas	A	PVP	2008	2011	7[a]
Vietnam	Social Health Insurance (SHI)	SHI	PVP	2003	2010	7
Ghana	National Health Insurance Scheme (NHIS)	SHI	PVP	2005	2008	3
Georgia	Medical Insurance Program (MIP)	A	PVP	2006	2011	5

Note: Thailand's UCS was created in 2002, building on the capacity of the Medical Service Welfare Program, which was created in 1975. Indonesia's Jamkesmas was created in 2008, building on the capacity created by its predecessor—the Askes created in 2004. In both cases the date of creation of the older program is used to measure "maturity". SHI in this table covers both the SHI+ and SHI++ models given in table 1.2. A = Autonomous; SHI = Embedded in SHI; PVP = Targeted to poor and vulnerable program; IS = Targeted to informal sector.
a. Maturity is defined as the length of time between the creation of the UHC program and the year of the household survey.

poor, others only a small fraction (figure 2.6). Thailand, Turkey, Colombia, Vietnam, and Peru have achieved the highest levels of enrollment of the poor, while Ghana, Georgia, and Indonesia had only managed to cover 30–40 percent of their poor. There is no clear correspondence between the degree of success with enrolling the poor and a certain "model:" the higher enrollment was obtained by countries using autonomous informal sector programs (Thailand and Colombia), embedded programs (Vietnam), autonomous poor and vulnerable (Peru), and a mix (Turkey). The countries with lower enrollment of the poor also include a mix of targeted poor and vulnerable programs (Georgia and Indonesia) and an embedded program (Ghana). In five of the eight countries, some of the poor were enrolled by UHC programs and some by a parallel SHI (indicated by shaded bars).

FIGURE 2.6
Enrollment of the Poor by Maturity of UHC Programs

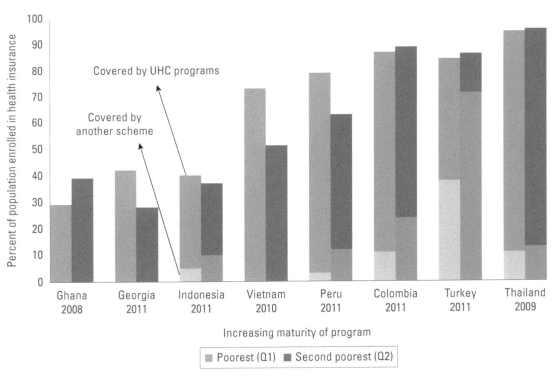

Sources: Colombia: Chernichovsky (2014); Georgia: World Bank (2012a); Ghana: NDPC (2009); Thailand: Limwattananon et al. (2012); Turkey: Atun et al. (2013); World Bank's calculation for Indonesia using National Socioeconomic Survey (Susenas), 2011; for Peru using National Household survey (ENAHO), 2011; and for Vietnam using Vietnam Household Living Standard Survey (VHLSS), 2010.
Note: The figure presents the countries in order of the "maturity" of the UHC programs, measured as the number of years between the creation of the program dealing with the poor and vulnerable and the year in which the household survey was carried out. It depicts enrollment of the poorest and second-poorest quintiles.

There is, however, an association between the maturity of the
program and success in enrolling the poor. The countries with the more
mature programs (Thailand, Turkey, Colombia, Peru, and Vietnam)
were more successful, while the countries with the younger programs
(Indonesia, Georgia, Ghana) had the lowest enrollment rates among
the poor.[8]

To illustrate enrollment of the nonpoor informal sector, in figure 2.7
we look at enrollment of the middle quintiles. In seven countries (including enrollment in the UHC program and other parallel programs), three
patterns stand out. Some countries have achieved high enrollment of all
quintiles (Thailand, Turkey, and Colombia); some have relatively high
coverage of the higher and lower quintiles (Vietnam and Peru), sometimes referred to as a "missing middle"; and some have generally lower
levels of enrollment at all levels, and enrollment is especially low for the
poorest quintiles (Ghana and Indonesia). For this third group, the most
distinctive feature is the "missing poor." As with enrollment of the poor,
the degree of success in enrolling the middle quintiles is associated with
program maturity.

FIGURE 2.7
Enrollment in Health Insurance by Income (All Schemes)

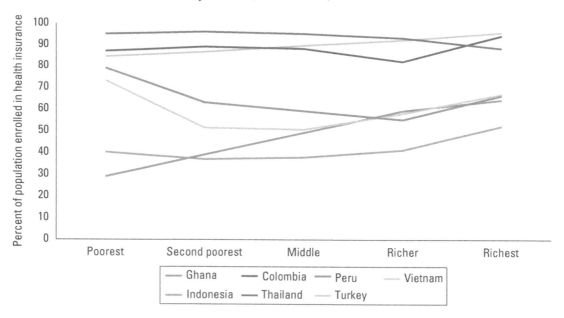

Sources: Colombia: Chernichovsky 2014; Ghana: NDPC 2009; Thailand: Limwattanagnon et al. 2012; Turkey: Atun et al. 2013;
Indonesia: authors' calculation using National Socioeconomic Survey (Susenas), 2011; Peru: World Bank's calculation using
National Household survey (ENAHO), 2011; and Vietnam: World Bank's calculation using Vietnam Household Living Standard
Survey (VHLSS), 2010.

Prioritizing Resources to the Poor

On the second intermediate objective, as expected, there is a pattern across models (figure 2.8). The targeted programs in Turkey, Peru, Georgia, and Indonesia allocate a larger fraction of the total enrollment to the poorer quintiles than the programs designed to include other populations in Ghana, Vietnam, Thailand, and Colombia.

Our interest is to assess if the poor are being left behind. For the programs aiming to include other populations, it is more appropriate to measure this by asking if these programs assign at least 20 percent of the program enrollment to the poorest 20 percent of the population. By this measure, we find that the programs of Colombia, Vietnam, and Thailand meet this test, and it is only the Ghana NHIS program which (in 2008) allocated less than 20 percent of the enrollment to the poorest 20 percent (and less than 40 percent of enrollment to the poorest 40 percent of the population). Still, we should bear in mind that Ghana's NHIS was the youngest program in the figure.

FIGURE 2.8
Distribution of Enrollment by Economic Quintile in Selected UHC Programs

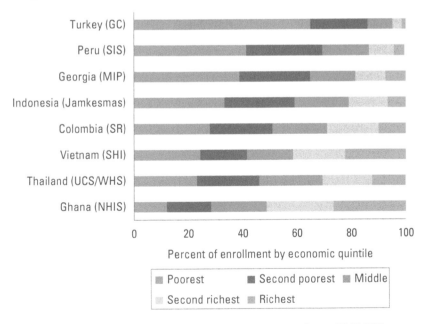

Sources: Colombia: Chernichovsky 2014; Georgia: World Bank 2012; Ghana: NDPC 2009; Thailand: Limwattanagnon et al. 2012; Turkey: Atun et al. 2013; Indonesia: authors' calculation using National Socioeconomic Survey (Susenas), 2011; Peru: World Bank's calculation using National Household survey (ENAHO), 2011; and Vietnam: World Bank's calculation using Vietnam Household Living Standard Survey (VHLSS), 2010.

In sum, all demand-side models can deliver high enrollment rates for the poor and for the nonpoor informal sector, and can achieve a minimum standard of targeting success. In other words, there is no "best model." Rather, success depends on quality of implementation, not on the choice of a certain model. We also find that maturity is associated with quality of implementation—the more mature programs have the best record on the intermediate objectives. Many reasons may explain this relationship, including maturity of institutions, maturity of policy, and development of a community of operators with required "UHC skills."

Conclusions and Policy Implications

After the year 2000, many developing countries used the opportunity provided by their newly developed capacities to identify and target people to attempt to change the prevailing pattern of regressive public expenditure in health by adopting a bottom-up approach to expand health coverage. This approach consists of the use of different strategies to reach different subpopulations, including the use of instruments designed to ensure that the poor and vulnerable do not get left behind. Countries following this approach combine the use of supply-side and demand-side programs to strengthen the coverage provided by the MoH. The former aim to reform and upgrade the production of health care services; these interventions often prioritize the poor and vulnerable through geographic targeting and through an emphasis on primary care and on services mostly utilized by the poor and vulnerable. The demand-side programs reduce the economic barriers to services for prioritized subpopulations, expanding their access to more and better services and to improved financial protection.

The demand-side programs are often launched with a first phase during which they are focused on targeting the poor and vulnerable; after a few years there is often a second phase when they expand their mandate to also include the nonpoor informal sector subpopulation. While the participation of the poor is always tax financed, the expansion to include the nonpoor informal sector can take two paths. Some countries follow a contributory path, which usually involves embedding the program within the SHI agencies. In this path, the informal sector can initially join the SHI program by making voluntary contributions. As the capacity to enforce the payment of contributions from this subpopulation increases, the participation of the informal sector becomes de facto mandatory. Countries following the noncontributory path create programs that operate autonomously from the SHI agencies and are mostly tax financed.

Below we summarize some implications for policy making and for research arising from these trends:

Targeting the Poor and Vulnerable

- *Implementation of the bottom-up approach is a viable option for developing countries.* Countries interested in pursuing a progressive path to expand health coverage should consider it.

- *Prioritizing the poor and vulnerable within a bottom-up approach may require ID and targeting capacities.* As countries improve the benefits, quality, and financial protection of publicly financed health care they can no longer rely on implicit targeting (that is, self-targeting by the better off) as when these programs were poorly resourced and unattractive. Countries seeking to implement a bottom-up approach are likely to have to develop capacity for explicit targeting.

- *To ensure that the ID and targeting systems are adapted for use by health programs, health policy makers should be participants in efforts to design them.*

- *Prioritizing the poor and vulnerable requires political leadership, as it often involves overcoming political obstacles during the transition to a bottom-up approach.*

Enrolling the Nonpoor Informal Sector

- *In countries with an SHI system, enrolling the nonpoor informal sector through a noncontributory tax-financed path has advantages and disadvantages.* A merit is that the expansion of coverage from the poor to the rest of the informal sector can be very rapid (given capacity of health care providers). A demerit is a trade-off between equity in the benefit package (comparing the autonomous program and the SHI) and fiscal sustainability (due to fiscal costs and increased informality). Resolving this trade-off may require deep tax and health reforms down the road to replace the mixed system by a fully tax-funded system.

- *Enrolling the informal sector through a mandatory contributory path presents fewer risks of sustainability but involves a slower pace in coverage expansion.* This is because it requires capacities to be built so as to identify incomes and collect contributions from the informal population.

- *Voluntary insurance is not a viable path to UHC.* It may, however, be a useful transitional stage while countries develop the capacity to move either to a mandatory contributory path or to a noncontributory tax-financed path.

Choosing a Model and a Path

- *There is no best practice model that can accommodate any country at any stage of development.* The best is one that corresponds to the socioeconomic fundamentals of the country, invests in the creation of the institutions and capacities required to manage the increasing complexity of the health system, and recognizes the need for frequent adaptation.

- *Socioeconomic fundamentals determine the viability of interventions.* While coverage of the poor and vulnerable has been achieved by low- and middle-income countries, the expansion to cover the nonpoor informal sector is more demanding of fiscal revenues and implementation capacity, and has generally been more successful in richer countries with smaller informal sectors, lower poverty ratios, and larger government revenues.

- *The road to UHC uses stepping stones, but they do not have to create path dependence.* Some of the institutions have a transitional role, such as targeting only the poor and the use of voluntary health insurance to cover the nonpoor informal sector. We found no evidence that the introduction of these institutions locked countries into a path or created path dependence. Countries that began UHC with targeted programs for the poor were able later to expand their coverage to other subpopulations. The road to UHC is long: choices made along that road may be suboptimal for a *final* configuration of the health system but appropriate for a system *in transition*.

Notes

1. This insight is also developed in Kutzin, Cashin, and Yip (forthcoming).
2. This configuration corresponds with the majority of UNICO countries, although the bottom-up approach and the findings of this chapter are also relevant for countries operating only with an MoH equivalent.
3. An exception to this is common in many Latin American countries, where SHI agencies often own and run their own hospitals, which operate as public hospitals except that they only accept SHI contributors as patients.
4. At an early stage in the development of targeting institutions, Gelbach and Pritchett (1999) argued provocatively that "more for the poor is less for the poor"; if policy makers ignore political feasibility they will choose full

targeting, thereby undermining political support from the middle class for the program they wish to finance, possibly leading to smaller budgets.

5. The term "TRs"—for which each country has its own name—is suggested by Robert Palacios (personal communication, December 2014) to distinguish these institutions from the large and growing number of systems for keeping official lists (of people or items).

6. For Thailand the findings were that UCS encouraged employment among married women but reduced formal-sector employment among married men, and increased informal sector employment among married women; the largest effect was in agriculture.

7. There also exist several studies that found no impact on informality. See World Bank 2012b for a careful review of the literature.

8. In Vietnam, the SHI was created in 1998, but the program for the poor was created only in 2002, so we consider the later date to measure "maturity." On the other hand, in Thailand, the UHC program was created in 2002, but it built on the experience of a much older program which targeted the poor, the Medical Welfare Scheme, which was created in 1975.

References

Aterido, Reyes, Mary Hallward-Driemeier, and Carmen Pages. 2011. "Does Expanding Health Insurance beyond Formal-Sector Workers Encourage Informality? Measuring the Impact of Mexico's Seguro Popular." Policy Research Working Paper 5785, World Bank and Inter-American Development Bank, Washington, DC.

Atun, R., S. Aydın, S. Chakraborty, S. Sümer, M. Aran, I. Gürol, S. Nazlıoğlu, S. Ozgülcü, U. Aydoğan, B. Ayar, U. Dilmen, and R. Akdağ. 2013. "Universal Health Coverage in Turkey: Enhancement of Equity." *The Lancet* 382 (9886): 65–99.

Besley, T., and S. M. Ravi Kanbur. 1990. "The Principles of Targeting." Working Paper 385, Office of the Vice President, Development Economics, World Bank, Washington, DC.

Bitran, Ricardo. 2014. "Universal Health Coverage and the Challenge of Informal Employment: Lessons from Developing Countries." Working Paper 87077, World Bank, Washington, DC.

Camacho, Adriana, Emily Conover, and Alejandro Hoyos. 2013. "Effects of Colombia's Social Protection System on Workers' Choice between Formal and Informal Employment." Policy Research Working Paper 6564, World Bank, Washington, DC.

Chernichovsky, Dov. 2014. "Disaggregating Private Healthcare Spending for Improved Policy: The Case of Colombia." PROESA, Cali, Colombia.

Cobham, Alex. 2005. "Tax Evasion, Tax Avoidance and Development Finance." *Queen Elizabeth House, Série documents de travail* 129.

Filmer, Deon. 2003. "The Incidence of Public Expenditures on Health and Education." Background note for World Development Report 2004: *Making Services Work for Poor People*, World Bank, Washington, DC.

Gelbach, Jonah B., and Lant H. Pritchett. 1999. "More for the Poor Is Less for the Poor: The Politics of Targeting." Policy Research Working Paper 1799, World Bank, Washington, DC.

Grosh, Margaret E., Carlo Del Ninno, Emil Tesliuc, and Azedine Ouerghi. 2008. *For Protection and Promotion: The Design and Implementation of Effective Safety Nets.* Washington, DC: World Bank.

Gwatkin, Davidson R., Adam Wagstaff, and Abdo Yazbeck, eds. 2005. *Reaching the Poor with Health, Nutrition, and Population Services: What Works, What Doesn't, and Why.* Washington, DC: World Bank.

ILO (International Labour Organization). 2013. *Key Indicators of the Labour Market.* 8th ed. Geneva.

INEI (Instituto Nacional de Estadística e Informática [National Institute of Statistics and Information]). 2011. *ENAHO 2011 (Encuesta Nacional de Hogares sobre Condiciones de Vida y Pobreza* [National Household Survey on Living Conditions and Poverty]). Lima, Peru. Retrieved April 9, 2014, from http://webinei.inei.gob.pe/anda_inei/index.php/catalog/195.

IMF (International Monetary Fund). 2014. World Economic Outlook: Legacies, Clouds, Uncertainties. Washington, DC.

Jack, William. 2001. "Social Investment Funds: An Organizational Approach to Improved Development Assistance." *The World Bank Research Observer* 16 (1): 109–24.

Knaul, Felicia Marie, Eduardo González-Pier, Octavio Gómez-Dantés, David García-Junco, Héctor Arreola-Ornelas, Mariana Barraza-Lloréns, Rosa Sandoval, Francisco Caballero, Mauricio Hernández-Avila, Mercedes Juan, David Kershenobich, Gustavo Nigenda, Enrique Ruelas, Jaime Sepúlveda, Roberto Tapia, Guillermo Soberón, Salomón Chertorivski, and Julio Frenk. 2012. "The Quest for Universal Health Coverage: Achieving Social Protection for All in Mexico." *The Lancet* 380 (9849): 1259–79.

Kutzin, Joseph, Cheryl Cashin, and Winnie Yip. Forthcoming. "Alternative Strategies for Universal Health Care Coverage." In *The Economics of Health and Health Systems.* Vol. 1 of *World Scientific Handbook of Global Health Economics and Public Policy,* edited by R. M. Scheffler. Singapore: World Scientific Publishing.

Levy, Santiago. 2008. *Good Intentions, Bad Outcomes: Social Policy, Informality, and Economic Growth in Mexico.* Washington, DC: Brookings Institution Press.

Limwattananon, Supon, Viroj Tangcharoensathien, Kanjana Tisayaticom, Tawekiat Boonyapaisarncharoen, and Phusit Prakongsai. 2012. "Why Has the Universal Coverage Scheme in Thailand Achieved a Pro-Poor Public Subsidy for Health Care?" *BMC Public Health* 12 (Suppl 1): S6.

Macinko, James. 2011. "A Preliminary Assessment of the Family Health Strategy in Brazil." World Bank, Washington, DC.

NDPC (National Development Planning Commission). 2009. *2008 Citizens' Assessment of the National Health Insurance Scheme: Towards a Sustainable Health Care Financing Arrangement That Protects the Poor.* Accra, Ghana: NDPC.

Saltman, Richard, Reinhard Busse, and Josep Figueras, eds. 2004. *Social Health Insurance Systems in Western Europe.* Maidenhead, UK: Open University Press.

Susenas (National Socio-Economic Survey). 2011. *Indonesia.* Jakarta: Central Bureau of Statistics (BPS).

Thornton, Rebecca L., Laurel E. Hatt, Erica M. Field, Mursaleena Islam, Freddy Solís Diaz, and Martha Azucena González. 2010. "Social Security Health Insurance for the Informal Sector in Nicaragua: A Randomized Evaluation." *Health Economics* 19 (S1): 181–206.

Towse, Adrian, Anne Mills, and Viroj Tangcharoensathien. 2004. "Learning from Thailand's Health Reforms." *BMJ: British Medical Journal* 328 (7431): 103.

Vietnam, General Statistics Office. 2012. *Result of the VHLSS (Vietnam Household Living Standard Survey) 2010.* Hanoi: General Statistics Office of Vietnam.

Wagstaff, Adam. 2014. "We Just Learned a Whole Lot More about Achieving Universal Health Coverage." *Let's Talk Development* (blog), August 25. http://blogs.worldbank.org/developmenttalk.

Wagstaff, Adam, and Wanwiphang Manachotphong. 2012. "Universal Health Care and Informal Labor Markets: The Case of Thailand." Policy Research Working Paper 6116, World Bank, Washington, DC.

World Bank. 2004. *World Development Report 2004: Making Services Work for Poor People.* Washington, DC: World Bank.

———. 2012a. *Georgia—Public Expenditure Review: Managing Expenditure Pressures for Sustainability and Growth.* Washington, DC: World Bank.

———. 2012b. "Mexico's System for Social Protection in Health and the Formal Sector." Human Development Department, Latin America and the Caribbean Regional Office, World Bank.

———. 2014. *World Development Indicators 2012.* Washington, DC: World Bank.

CHAPTER 3

Expanding Benefits: Exercising Choices to Expand the Scope of Health Care Services

To reiterate: Universal health coverage (UHC) aims to provide all people with access to needed health care services (including prevention, promotion, treatment, and rehabilitation) of the requisite quality to be effective, and without exposing the person to financial hardship (WHO 2010). Central to this definition is the provision of needed health care services, incorporating the nebulous concept of "need" that does not lend itself to easy measurement or even a standard application or interpretation. Kutzin (2013) interprets needed health care services as a component of effective coverage (chapter 5), breaking the former into two components—that all those who need a health intervention are aware of their need, and that all users who are aware of their need are able to demand and use the services they require.

UHC initiatives therefore aim to reduce the gap between the need and utilization of health care services. The pathways to UHC envisage progressing beyond the current coverage of health care services and eventually expanding into a comprehensive range of services that can effectively deliver interventions of requisite quality to address the health care needs of the covered population, as far as possible given the resources available.

While conceptual clarity on needed health services is in itself very helpful, health policy makers require much more information and guidance to achieve progress in their countries on the services or depth dimension of the UHC cube (chapter 1). In a context in which resources will always be limited vis-à-vis the very wide spectrum of potentially available health services, policy makers need to sift through and choose their coverage goal. But once that goal becomes clearer, they will still face

67

innumerable combinations of context-specific starting points and options for incremental coverage.

Measuring where a country stands on coverage of health services (or its benefit package) *at a given time* against the optimal service coverage goal required for it to qualify as UHC is also much more challenging than, say, measuring the share of population covered by the same program. The denominator of needed health services would tend to change with rising citizen expectations, improving health technology, and increasing ability to pay. Keeping this denominator practical and measurable is part of the measurement challenge, and is vital for monitoring progress in health service coverage. One recent framework for measuring progress toward UHC developed jointly by WHO and the World Bank (WHO and IBRD/World Bank 2014) applied the filters of relevance, quality, and availability to help countries select "tracer" indicators for prevention and treatment services.

There is also the central dilemma of prioritizing a benefit package when multiple objectives could pull policy makers in different directions, forcing them to trade off (table 3.1). The incorporation of the economic benefits of financial protection may add to the economic rationale for curative services, including clinic-based PHC and hospital-based care. Nor is it just the economic and public health criteria but often the political economy of the country that determines the choices made in designing benefit packages.

Thus in this UHC dimension of covered health care services, policy makers have to decide on numerous areas in expanding coverage.

TABLE 3.1
Relative Priorities and Trade-offs under Different Approaches to Expanding the Benefit Package

Priority	Traditional public health	PHC, clinic based	Hospital-based care
Status quo (varies widely)	Low	Low	High
Alma Ata (ideal)	High	High	Low
Alma Ata (real)	Low	High	Low
Economic efficiency	High	Low	High
Economic rationale (efficiency and equity)	Higher	Varies	Not so high
Full public sector rationale (efficiency, equity, and implementability)	Highest	Low	High

Source: Reproduced from Filmer, Hammer, and Pritchett 2002.

Given their sometimes very different starting points and multiple options for incremental additions, they naturally seek evidence and guidance to help them set the coverage goals—the spectrum of services that should eventually be covered to achieve effectiveness—to walk them through the practical considerations of what implementation involves. They may therefore benefit from the experiences of the 24 countries in the Universal Health Coverage Studies Series (UNICO) study.

Those experiences form the bedrock of this chapter, showing how the UNICO countries are adding services and going beyond the millennium development goals (MDGs); trending toward explicit benefit packages; using complex mechanisms in setting priorities for these packages; adopting, de facto, benefit packages smaller than promised; and generally shifting to closed-ended provider-payment mechanisms with improved linkages to performance. All are summed up in the final section, alongside suggested areas for further research.

Adding Services—Moving Beyond the MDGs

Based on the services added to plug gaps in coverage relative to the optimal service coverage goal, we classify the 26 UHC programs in three broad groups (table 3.2). The first batch of seven programs kept their focus on services related to the MDGs, and often complemented the health system's MDG services by adding other primary care services, such as those for noncommunicable diseases (NCDs). The second group of four (two of them in India) did not include any MDG-related services. As the MDG services were already provided by the broader health system, the programs were designed to cover new services beyond the usual health system focus on MDGs, such as hospitalization for secondary and tertiary care (RSBY and RA in India, respectively), drugs for chronic diseases (Jamaica), and curative coverage for HIV-related conditions (South Africa). The third category, the largest with 15 programs, had elements of both the previous categories. Most of the UNICO countries embarked on their UHC programs after establishing a relatively sound foundation of PHC services, especially those related to MDGs.

Table 3.3 shows how the 24 countries fared on financing and implementing tracer programs, each representing a commonly provided PHC service catering to communicable diseases, child health, maternal care, and NCDs.

MDG-related services, represented by the first three columns (communicable diseases, child health, and maternal care) are well established in most countries. They are population-based, using lists of named individuals or households to monitor compliance in two-thirds of the

TABLE 3.2

Trends in Adding Services Exemplified by the UHC Programs, 2011–12

Country	Maternity	Public health care services, such as immunizations	Outpatient primary care contacts	Hospital component	Dialysis or transplants	Program coverage summary
UHC focuses on and complements MDG services provided by the health system						
Argentina	Yes	Yes	Yes	No	No	MDG, Primary
Brazil	No	Yes	Yes	No	No	MDG, Primary
Ethiopia	Yes	Yes	Yes	No	No	MDG, Primary
Guatemala	No	Yes	Yes	No	No	MDG, Primary
India—NRHM	Yes	Yes	Yes	Yes	No	MDG, Primary
Kenya	No	Yes	No	No	No	MDG
Nigeria	Yes	Yes	Yes	No	No	MDG, Primary
The broader health system provides MDG services; the UHC program excludes MDG services, going beyond them						
India—RA	No	No	No	Yes	Yes	Hospital
India—RSBY	Yes	No	No	Yes	No	Hospital
Jamaica	n.a.	n.a.	n.a.	n.a.	n.a.	Primary
South Africa	No	Yes	Yes	Yes	Yes	Primary and Hospital for HIV
UHC complements MDG services and adds inpatient services—elements of both previous categories						
Chile	Yes	No	Yes	Yes	Yes	MDG, Primary, Hospital
China	Yes	Yes	Yes and No	Yes	No	MDG, Primary, Hospital
Colombia	Yes	Yes	Yes	Yes	Yes	MDG, Primary, Hospital
Costa Rica	Yes	Yes	Yes	Yes	Yes	MDG, Primary, Hospital
Georgia	Yes	No	Yes	Yes	No	MDG, Primary, Hospital
Ghana	Yes	n.a.	No	Yes	No	MDG, Primary, Hospital
Indonesia	Yes	Yes	Yes	Yes	Yes	MDG, Primary, Hospital

table continues next page

TABLE 3.2 *(Continued)*

Country	Maternity	Public health care services, such as immunizations	Outpatient primary care contacts	Hospital component	Dialysis or transplants	Program coverage summary
Kyrgyz Republic	Yes	Yes	Yes	Yes	Yes	MDG, Primary, Hospital
Mexico	Yes	Yes	Yes	Yes	Yes	MDG, Primary, Hospital
Philippines	Yes	Yes	Yes	Yes	Yes	MDG, Primary, Hospital
Peru	Yes	Yes	Yes	Yes	No	MDG, Primary, Hospital
Thailand	Yes	Yes	Yes	Yes	Yes	MDG, Primary, Hospital
Tunisia	Yes	Yes	Yes	Yes	Yes	MDG, Primary, Hospital
Turkey	Yes	Yes	Yes	Yes	Yes	MDG, Primary, Hospital
Vietnam	Yes	Yes	Yes	Yes	Yes	MDG, Primary, Hospital

Source: UNICO studies.
Note: n.a. = not applicable.

TABLE 3.3
Financing and Implementation of Primary Care Programs (% of UNICO countries)

	Communicable diseases (tracer: TB)	Child health (tracer: routine immunization)	Maternal care (tracer: maternity services)	NCDs (tracer: diabetes)
Has earmarked funding from central source	65	66	66	27
Requires copayment by user	4	12	12	48
Often requires informal payments	7	7	30	22
Health workers use a population-based list of names to monitor program implementation	58	66	63	28
Use of technical protocols is effectively enforced in most primary care clinics	71	75	74	39
Reports for previous year have been published based on administrative data	88	91	95	43

Source: UNICO studies.
Note: These represent UNICO countries as a whole and not just UHC programs in these countries.

countries; have developed technical protocols and these protocols are generally used in most primary care clinics in three-fourths of the countries; report regularly on their activities and on progress toward targets in 90 percent of countries; and have secure funding sources.

These MDG-related services do not require formal or informal copayments from patients (with very few exceptions), and although maternity services seem weaker than communicable diseases and child health programs, most case studies indicate that they are also relatively strong. Most UNICO countries now have programs to exempt maternity services from user fees (71 percent) and a third of the countries subsidize transport for deliveries. However, problems exist on quality assurance of providers and on access to emergency obstetric care, including safe blood transfusions.

In contrast, coverage for NCDs (increasingly the bulk of the disease burden in these countries—table 3.6 below) remains much weaker than for MDG-related services. Financing, exemptions from user fees, and protection from out-of-pocket expenditure (OOPE) on drugs and other services, monitoring, and use of protocols are generally far less developed. It is no wonder that many of the new-millennium UHC programs are beginning to focus on reducing this persistent, wide gap through plans to better cover NCDs.

UNICO Countries' Initial Actions toward UHC—Generally Aligned with Current Recommendations

Recent publications on this subject seem to endorse the directional approach taken by the UNICO countries. The Lancet Commission on Global Health 2035 (Jamison et al. 2013) acknowledges trade-offs that may arise between the two key focus areas of UHC programs—health outcomes and financial protection—and suggested two pathways to expand benefit packages in what the authors term "progressive universalism." In the first, they suggest tax-funded coverage for the entire population with a pro-poor benefit package that includes infectious diseases, reproductive and child health care services, and essential NCD and injury coverage. The concept of a pro-poor benefit package suggests that, at least to some extent, targeting could be achieved through the contents of benefit packages (though more research is needed). In the second, they suggest a combination of financing modalities making for a larger benefit package, exempting the poor from any contributions, but requiring greater administrative effort to identify and exempt them. The Lancet Commission suggests coverage for high-cost interventions only along this progressive pathway to

UHC, appreciating that most (though not all) high-cost interventions provide low value for money on intended health outcomes and on financial protection.

A WHO consultative group on equity and UHC (WHO 2014) suggested a three-pronged strategy for countries seeking fair and equitable progress toward UHC: categorizing services into priority classes, using criteria such as cost-effectiveness, priority of services needed by the poor, and financial risk protection; starting with coverage expansion for high-priority services to everyone (similar to one of the above Lancet Commission pathways); and ensuring inclusiveness for disadvantaged groups, such as the poor and those living in rural areas.

This emerging global convergence of advice on prioritizing expansion of UHC parallels UNICO countries' own experience over the last decade or so. Almost all the UNICO countries initially prioritized coverage for cost-effective and pro-poor interventions, such as maternity services and immunization (also prioritized under the MDGs), which were always covered under their UHC programs or otherwise through the country's health system. This was not always true, however, for essential NCD and injury coverage.

Beyond the MDGs

Based on the MDG package of maternal, child health, and infectious disease services as the most common starting point or early priority, the next expansion was usually for coverage to include outpatient primary care. Though again widespread in overall adoption, this growth showed variations, often reflecting national income and revealing how resources guided it (table 3.4 is arranged by the order of increasing gross domestic product (GDP) per capita in 2011, to illustrate this aspect). Almost all countries offering such outpatient primary care services also extended coverage to pharmaceuticals, laboratory and basic radiology services, and specialist consultations.

Not quite as common, two-thirds of countries with outpatient care covered higher-end diagnostic imaging. Again, per capita GDP was important: almost all higher-income countries offered coverage for inpatient services, but only one of the three low-income countries did. Where available, such coverage generally included physician service components, pharmaceuticals, and basic and higher-end diagnostic imaging.

Coverage for wage loss due to health events such as sickness or maternity was only available in a small proportion of UHC programs, mainly in the middle-income countries. This is unsurprising, as wage loss compensation is often a costly proposition (and prone to moral hazard) linked to

TABLE 3.4
Summary of the Content of Benefit Packages in UNICO Countries, 2011

Country	Maternity	Emergency services	Hospital services	Physician service components	Pharmaceuticals	Public health services, e.g. immunization	Outpatient primary care	Outpatient specialist care
Ethiopia	Yes	No	No	No	No	Yes	Yes	No
Kenya	No	No	No	No	No	Yes	No	No
Kyrgyz Republic	Yes	Yes	Yes	Yes	Yes	Yes	Yes	Yes
India—RA	No	Yes	Yes	Yes	Yes	No	No	No
India—RSBY	Yes	Yes	Yes	Yes	Yes	No	No	No
India—NRHM	Yes	Yes	Yes	Yes	Yes	Yes	Yes	Yes
Vietnam	Yes	Yes	Yes	Yes	Yes	Yes	Yes	Yes
Ghana	Yes	Yes	Yes	Yes	Yes	n/a	No	Yes
Philippines	Yes	n/a	Yes	Yes	Yes	Yes	Yes	Yes
Nigeria	Yes	Yes	No	No	No	Yes	Yes	Yes
Georgia	Yes	Yes	Yes	Yes	Yes	No	Yes	Yes
Guatemala	No	No	No	No	No	Yes	Yes	No
Indonesia	Yes	Yes	Yes	Yes	Yes	Yes	Yes	Yes
Tunisia	Yes	Yes	Yes	Yes	Yes	Yes	Yes	Yes
Thailand	Yes	Yes	Yes	Yes	Yes	Yes	Yes	Yes
Jamaica	n/a	n/a	n/a	n/a	n/a	n/a	n/a	n/a
China	Yes	Yes	Yes	Yes	Yes	Yes	Yes and No	Yes and No
Peru	Yes	Yes	Yes	Yes and No	Yes	Yes	Yes	Yes
Colombia	Yes	Yes	Yes	Yes	Yes	Yes	Yes	Yes
South Africa	No	No	Yes	Yes	Yes	Yes	Yes	Yes
Costa Rica	Yes	Yes	Yes	Yes	Yes	Yes	Yes	Yes
Mexico	Yes	Yes	Yes	Yes	Yes	Yes	Yes	Yes
Turkey	Yes	Yes	Yes	Yes	Yes	Yes	Yes	Yes
Brazil	No	No	No	No	No	Yes	Yes	No
Argentina	Yes	Yes	No	No	No	Yes	Yes	Yes
Chile	Yes	Yes	Yes	Yes	Yes	No	Yes	Yes

Source: UNICO studies.
Note: Countries are sorted according to their GDP per capita (current US$) as of year 2011; n/a = not available.

Pharmaceuticals for outpatient	Clinical lab tests for outpatient services	Imaging for outpatient - basic (X rays and ultrasound)	Diagnostic imaging beyond basic (e.g. MRI, CT Scan)	Eyeglasses	Mental health/ behavioral	Dialysis or Transplants	GDP per capita (current USD, 2011)
No	No	No	No	No	No	No	351
Yes	No	No	No	No	No	No	816
Yes	Yes	Yes	Yes	No	Yes	Yes	1,124
No	No	No	No	No	No	Yes	1,540
No	No	No	No	No	No	No	1,540
Yes	Yes	Yes	No	No	Yes	No	1,540
Yes	Yes	Yes	Yes	No	Yes	Yes	1,543
Yes	Yes	Yes	Yes	No	No	No	1,594
No	Yes	Yes	No	No	No	Yes	2,358
Yes	Yes	Yes	No	No	Yes	No	2,519
Yes	No	Yes	No	No	No	No	3,220
No	No	No	No	No	No	No	3,240
Yes	Yes	Yes	Yes	Yes	Yes	Yes	3,470
Yes	Yes	Yes	Yes	No	Yes	Yes	4,305
Yes	Yes	Yes	Yes	Yes	Yes	Yes	5,192
n/a	n/a	n/a	n/a	n/a	n/a	n/a	5,346
Yes and No	Yes and No	Yes and No	Yes and No	No	No	No	5,447
Yes	Yes	Yes	Yes	Yes	No	No	5,759
Yes	Yes	Yes	Yes	Yes	Yes	Yes	7,125
Yes	Yes	No	No	No	Yes	Yes	7,831
Yes	Yes	Yes	Yes	Yes	Yes	Yes	8,704
Yes	Yes	Yes	Yes	No	Yes	Yes	9,803
Yes	Yes	Yes	Yes	Yes	Yes	Yes	10,605
No	Yes	No	No	No	Yes	No	12,576
No	Yes	Yes	Yes	No	No	No	13,694
Yes	Yes	Yes	Yes	Yes	Yes	Yes	14,511

the country's paying capacity for welfare programs, and has linkages to the degree of formal sector development and its participation in the UHC program (where wages are known or easier to determine).

Defining Benefits—Toward Explicit Benefit Packages

Even as countries get richer, health care needs expand more than the resources available, forcing policy makers to decide which health care services can be adequately covered—and which cannot. One of their main tools—benefit packages—can be described in many ways: for example, by the level of health care services covered (combinations of coverage for primary, secondary, or tertiary care, or comprehensive coverage, encompassing all levels of care); by the specific services covered (maternal and child health, family planning services, screening and/or case management for NCDs, and the like); or by how they are defined (including explicit benefit packages). This section focuses on the third: how the UNICO countries define their increasingly explicit benefit packages.

Policy makers' responses to the funding–coverage dilemma can be broken down as follows (Giedion, Bitran, and Tristao 2014):

- *Implicit rationing.* No restrictions are expressly laid out and so most or even all services are possible in theory, but are not really available. This may be due to authorization requirements, delayed care or waiting lists, care denied at point of service (pharmaceutical stockouts or nonavailability, for instance), or dilution of care through incomplete services. Many of the UNICO countries have had such systems in the past or these systems exist parallel to the UHC programs even today.

- *Implicit rationing combined with systematic priority setting processes and other strategies.* In this more evolved policy response (exemplified by the United Kingdom), implicit rationing coexists with proactive strategies for priority setting, review of evidence, and evaluation of health care services' cost-effectiveness.

- *Explicit benefit packages.* Services to be covered (or excluded) are explicitly defined, often via positive and negative lists. Positive lists— where all covered services are explicitly listed and everything else not listed is not covered by the program—reflect benefit packages becoming increasingly explicit. Negative lists mean that all health care services other than those in the list are part of the benefit package, which also implies automatic coverage for new drugs, diagnostic imaging, and procedures (unless they eventually find their way into the negative list). As benefit packages become more explicit, even where implicit rationing is used, positive lists often cover drug benefits; negative lists are becoming longer.

Positive lists come in various types: coverage by health conditions (diagnosis-based), clinical procedures (procedure-based), a listing for covered drugs, and sometimes specific population groups. Very few UNICO countries, however, used standardized coding systems such as ICD[1] for diagnosis or any of the procedure coding systems to specify the exact coverage. Indonesia (with ICD-9) and Turkey (with ICD-10) have attempted this, which may help support future reform options to use payment systems such as diagnosis-related groups (DRGs)—see *Contracting Benefits* below.

All but three UNICO programs (Costa Rica, India—NRHM, and Tunisia) use explicit benefit packages to move from the implicit rationing often inherent in the broad, but often overambitious, promises in their implicit benefit packages (see *Breaking Promises* below). Most of them explicitly define their benefit packages via positive lists or a combination of positive and negative lists (table 3.5). Some of the countries using

TABLE 3.5
Explicit Benefit Packages in UNICO countries, 2011–12

Country and program	Description
Argentina—Plan Nacer	Positive list: Combines health conditions, clinical procedures, and other broad categories.
Brazil—Primary Health Care Extension Strategy (PHCES)	Positive list: Health conditions and clinical procedures, ICD-10 codes not used.
Chile—AUGE	Positive list of prioritized health problems, further detailed as a set of guaranteed services with their protocols.
Costa Rica—CCSS	Not explicit: Only broad categories. However, for pharmaceuticals, negative list exists.
Georgia—MIP	Positive and negative lists: Broad categories of services included, and also some explicit exclusions.
Ghana—NHIS	Negative list: Comprehensive benefit package with an exclusion list.
Guatemala—PEC	Positive list: Health conditions (and population groups).
India—NRHM, RA, and RSBY	Not explicit in NRHM, positive list in RA and positive and negative lists in RSBY. ICD-10 codes are not used.

table continues next page

TABLE 3.5 *(Continued)*

Country and program	Description
Indonesia—Jamkesmas	Positive and negative lists: Structured as a list of inclusions and exclusions. Defined by health conditions, clinical procedures and other broad categories. For health conditions, ICD-9 codes are used.
Jamaica—NHF	Positive list of NCD drugs to be covered under the program. The benefit package is defined by health conditions and broad categories based on doctors certifications.
Kenya—HSSF	Explicit. Kenya's HSSF package is structured by broad categories, which include age cohorts, and by detailed categories, which are defined by the Kenya Essential Package of Health Services. No ICD-10 codes are used though.
Kyrgyz Republic—SGBP	*Positive list:* The benefit package has a positive list, by health condition (DRGs), for inpatient care, and also for drugs in outpatient care settings. Coverage for outpatient care is otherwise defined by level of care.
Mexico—Seguro Popular	*Several Positive lists:* CAUSES (Comisión Nacional de Protección Social en Salud) covering first- and second-level care—275 Interventions. FPGC (Consejo de Salubridad General)—57 interventions in 16 diseases (high-cost treatment). SMNG (insurance for children)—128 additional interventions.
Nigeria—NHIS-MDG-MCH/MSS/MPHC in Ondo State	The project benefit package is defined by health conditions for pregnant women and for children under 5 years. There are no ICD-10 codes used.
Peru—SIS	Has an explicitly defined benefit package, structured mostly by health conditions (both as a positive and a negative list).
Philippines—Sponsored Program for Poor Families (SP)	Positive and negative lists. It has lists of clinical procedures and health conditions covered (such as TB, cataract surgery, malaria, pregnancy.). It also has a negative list of excluded services.
South Africa—ATP	Positive list, by health conditions and by clinical procedures, including laboratory testing for HIV. Individuals who are assessed as HIV positive with a CD4 count below 350 cells/mm^3 are entitled. Pregnant women and individuals with TB are enrolled regardless of CD4 count. No ICD-10 codes used though.
Thailand—UCS	Positive and negative lists: An explicitly defined benefit package structured as a list of inclusions and exclusions. The benefit package is defined by health conditions, clinical procedures, and other broad and detailed categories. No ICD codes are used.
Tunisia—FMAP	*Not explicit:* There is no benefit package defined in the public facilities, and it is an implicit package determined by technological ability of the specific health care providers.
Turkey—Green Card	*Positive List:* It has an explicitly defined benefit package structured as an inclusion list. The benefit package is defined by health conditions, clinical procedures, and other broad and detailed categories. It also uses ICD-10 codes.
Vietnam—SHI	*Positive and negative lists:* The benefit package is defined as a list of health services covered and a negative list of explicitly excluded services. The package is defined by clinical procedures and other broad categories of benefits, sometimes specifying additional conditions under which the benefit is covered (for example transportation costs only covered for the poor). ICD-10 or other standardized coding system is not used.

Source: UNICO studies.

positive lists also provide for coverage exclusions within the defined scope of cover through negative lists. It is often politically harder to make exclusions known and explicit, but explicit packages can help flag the need for the resources to deliver the services and to organize them, auguring well for actual delivery of the promised package.

For comparison, almost all European Union (EU) countries use positive lists though very often only for drugs and less often for covered medical procedures. Only a minority use implicit rationing and have only negative lists (Paris, Devaux, and Wei 2010).

Prioritizing Services—Mechanics and Complexities

The above UNICO trends suggest that prioritizing the services for initial coverage—and for adding to existing services—is an important decision area for health financing programs. Prioritization helps compel decisions on more effective services than those of questionable value, helps reclarify criteria for allocating scarce resources, and makes these decisions transparent, often involving consultations with stakeholders and incorporating their views (Wong and Bitran 1999). Policy makers committed to systematic prioritization require detailed information and a good understanding of their options on the institutional structure, processes, and criteria to be used.

Institutional Mechanism

Their first important decision is on the institutional mechanism for prioritizing services for initial UHC program coverage. In most Organisation for Economic Co-operation and Development (OECD) countries, as increasingly higher health expenditures are allocated to new drugs and technology, decisions on these services are delegated more and more to specialized bodies (Landwehr and Bohm 2011). Specialized agencies can make these decisions more easily and in an apolitical, scientific, and credible manner (Flinders 2008), because, for example, countries using negative lists to define their benefit package will find it unpopular to add to the list. Still, these agencies need built-in safeguards to prevent a potential loss of accountability (Landwehr and Bohm 2011).

A related issue, when establishing the institutional mechanisms for prioritizing, is the extent and nature of stakeholder involvement, which could potentially include that of public and provider representatives. While such involvement can improve buy-in and legitimacy, it also needs to be weighed against a possible increase in transaction costs, greater difficulty in arriving at decisions (Landwehr and Bohm 2011), and the risk of interested stakeholders "capturing" the consultation process (Coen and Thatcher 2005).

A compromise pathway is often adopted: allowing stakeholders a greater say in defining the principles and criteria to be used, and then leaving it to the specialized bodies to make the decisions in a scientific, accountable, and transparent manner. The WHO consultative group on equity and UHC (WHO 2014) suggests that priorities must be set based on scientific evidence, ethical arguments, and public values. To properly integrate these elements, it stressed the importance of explicit, systematic, and continuous processes for priority setting and use of a health technology assessment (HTA).[2] Countries such as Australia, Colombia, Denmark, Finland, Germany, Mexico, the Netherlands, New Zealand, Norway, Sweden, Thailand, the United Kingdom, and the United States have extensively used techniques such as HTA. Thailand has also sought to integrate elements of direct public participation in its HTA process.

Criteria for Setting Priorities and Amending Them

The next decision area requires the criteria for priority setting and subsequent amendments to the benefit package to be defined, in tune with the objectives of the UHC program. The criteria could range from the country's disease profile and burden—for its vulnerable groups particularly—to evidence from scientific and systematic cost-effectiveness studies and HTAs. Such criteria need to try to meet the twin objectives of adequate financial protection for vulnerable groups and sustainability for the program. However, the role played by the cultural context and political economy can be paramount (an expression of a society's values that may differ from another's), and may explain why the pathways to UHC vary.

In the UNICO countries, affordability[3] and cost-effectiveness were the commonest criteria for defining the benefit packages (box 3.1), but in half the programs studied no formal criteria were specified. The emphasis on cost-effectiveness appears not just a desirable stated by respondents but also a reality evidenced by the content of the packages. Some of the public health interventions known as the most cost-effective are offered by almost all studied programs, more commonly than outpatient, inpatient, or wage-loss elements of benefit packages (see previous section). However, as we move along the continuum of what is added beyond these public health interventions, choices made for outpatient and inpatient coverage may not always be based on cost-effectiveness. In the real world, political economy factors—such as the

---

BOX 3.1
Criteria for Defining Benefit Packages

Via the questionnaire (appendix D), the UNICO study collected and analyzed information on the common criteria used to define benefit packages by the 26 programs. The commonest were affordability (17 programs), cost-effectiveness (15), financial protection (14), opinion of scientific community (13), and no criteria formally specified (6).

Most of the programs did not, however, systematically determine affordability. The majority drew up their initial budget for the package with reference to what the government was willing to spend, some-times also using benchmarking or even best guesswork; only a minority conducted actuarial analysis (box 4.1), systematic estimation of costs, formal cost-effectiveness study, or HTA. This vagueness led the SIS program in Peru, for example, into a major mismatch between what it promised and what it could feasibly achieve.

This seemingly unscientific approach may not necessarily reflect policy makers' unwillingness to consider evidence. It may instead reflect lack of tools, know-how, and global evidence, underscoring the need for systematic work on identifying and prioritizing affordable interventions for different contexts along lines of country income, burden of disease, and health expenditure patterns, etc.

"rescue principle" for conditions with high visibility[4]—influence decisions. An example of such a program in the UNICO cases is the RA program in India, which focuses on high-cost, tertiary care. (Examining which of these prioritization criteria change or become increasingly important as benefit packages expand, or as country income grows, requires further research.)

Among UNICO countries, causes of the overall disease burden varied widely by income and region, with some notable exceptions such as Georgia and South Africa. As in most countries globally, NCDs were predominant causes of morbidity and mortality in UNICO countries, accounting for more than 75 percent of all disability-adjusted life years (DALYs) lost in Argentina, Chile, China, Costa Rica, Georgia, and Turkey. Communicable diseases dominated the disease burden in Sub-Saharan African countries, including Ethiopia, Ghana, Kenya, Nigeria, and South Africa (table 3.6). Ischemic heart disease was the biggest cause of the disease burden in nine of 24 UNICO countries; lower respiratory tract infections in five countries; HIV/AIDS in four; and stroke three. Interpersonal violence was the largest cause of DALYs in Colombia; malaria was prominent in Ghana; and diabetes dominated the disease burden in Mexico.

Revisions to benefit packages in UNICO countries are rarely accompanied by an assessment of fiscal impact and budget availability (table 3.7),

TABLE 3.6
Overall Burden of Disease in UNICO Countries, 2010

Country	Share of burden of disease (%)			Top three causes of burden of disease		
	NCDs	CDs	Injuries	#1	#2	#3
Argentina	76	13	11	Ischemic heart disease	Stroke	Major depressive disorder
Brazil	69	17	15	Ischemic heart disease	Interpersonal violence	Low back pain
Chile	79	9	13	Ischemic heart disease	Low back pain	Stroke
China	77	10	13	Stroke	Ischemic heart disease	Chronic obstructive pulmonary disease
Colombia	61	21	18	Interpersonal violence	Ischemic heart disease	Major depressive disorder
Costa Rica	77	12	12	Ischemic heart disease	Major depressive disorder	Low back pain
Ethiopia	28	63	9	Lower respiratory infections	Diarrheal diseases	Malaria
Georgia	81	11	8	Ischemic heart disease	Stroke	Chronic obstructive pulmonary disease
Ghana	34	60	6	Malaria	HIV/AIDS	Lower respiratory infections
Guatemala	46	37	17	Lower respiratory infections	Interpersonal violence	Diarrheal diseases
India	45	43	12	Preterm birth complications	Diarrheal diseases	Lower respiratory infections
Indonesia	58	33	9	Stroke	Tuberculosis	Road injury
Jamaica	64	23	13	HIV/AIDS	Diabetes	Stroke
Kenya	24	69	7	HIV/AIDS	Lower respiratory infections	Malaria
Kyrgyz Republic	58	29	13	Ischemic heart disease	Lower respiratory infections	Stroke
Mexico	71	15	13	Diabetes	Ischemic heart disease	Chronic kidney disease
Nigeria	20	71	9	Lower respiratory infections	HIV/AIDS	Lower respiratory infections
Peru	62	28	10	Lower respiratory infections	Major depressive disorder	Ischemic heart disease
Philippines	58	33	9	Lower respiratory infections	Ischemic heart disease	Tuberculosis
South Africa	31	61	9	HIV/AIDS	Diarrheal diseases	Interpersonal violence
Thailand	66	19	14	HIV/AIDS	Ischemic heart disease	Road injury
Tunisia	72	16	12	Ischemic heart disease	Road injury	Major depressive disorder
Turkey	76	16	8	Ischemic heart disease	Stroke	Major depressive disorder
Vietnam	66	21	13	Stroke	Road injury	Low back pain

Source: Murray et al. 2013.

TABLE 3.7

Prioritization Process and Criteria for Creating and Revising Benefit Packages, Selected UNICO Countries, 2012

Country and program	Process and criteria for prioritizing
Argentina—Plan Nacer	Revised annually by the national Ministry of Health (MoH). No individual explicit criteria; however, must target infant and maternal mortality and consider budgetary concerns.
Brazil—PHCES	Set and revised by the MoH and the state and municipal health secretariats (Council of State Health Secretaries). No explicit and formally required criteria. Loosely assessed cost-effectiveness evidence and financial protection considerations play a role.
Chile—AUGE	AUGE Consultative Committee in the MoH defines and revises the package. Prioritization includes an algorithm to consider burden of disease, epidemiological significance, share of the population suffering, expected cost per beneficiary, supply capacity, and effectiveness of interventions, etc.
Costa Rica—CCSS	No formal processes for modification, though regulations establish that the services will be provided within the financial capacity of the CCSS. For pharmaceuticals, the unit of pharmaco-epidemiology uses cost-effectiveness and opinions of scientific community as criteria to define its policies. It plans to develop an HTA group in the future.
Georgia—MIP	Defined by the MoH. No criteria are formally specified for including benefits. Budget parameters implicitly affect the benefits. The scientific community has very little involvement.
Ghana—NHIS	Originally, a task force developed an exclusion package, based on scientific discussions. There has been no revision to the package and no criteria formally specified for inclusion of benefits. Any modification of the package is expected to take into account fiscal impact and budget availability and estimated premium rates based on actuarial analysis, even though premiums may then have to be subsidized.
Guatemala—PEC	Originally set by MoH technical experts with support from Inter-American Development Bank consultants. The criteria were based on cost-effective interventions and expert opinions on acceptability and relevance.
India—NRHM, RSBY, and RA	Benefit packages are usually designed and updated by the administrative department/s implementing the program. They usually consult with the medical community when designing or updating the packages.
Indonesia—Jamkesmas	The MoH has the mandate to revise and set the package, but no process or criteria are formally specified. Jamkesmas' package was based on the existing package for the Civil Servants Social Health Insurance (Askes) and therefore did not formally use criteria such as cost-effectiveness. One significant revision to the package was in 2008 when the drug formulary was introduced, mainly generic drugs, again adapted from Askes. Experience suggests that budget availability is taken into account for package modification.
Jamaica—NHF	The Medical Committee—doctors and pharmacists—reviews the drug list and its reimbursement rates, and makes recommendations. The criteria for inclusion of benefits include cost-effectiveness and affordability, and the scientific community's opinion.

table continues next page

TABLE 3.7 *(Continued)*

Country and program	Process and criteria for prioritizing
Kenya—HSSF	The benefit package was designed taking into account the evaluation that was carried out by Kenya Medical Research Institute (KEMRI) Welcome Trust. The criteria for inclusion of benefits relate fully to cost-effectiveness; all the services included in the Kenya Basic Health package supported by the UHC program are evidence based and cost effective. Affordability, financial protection, and the scientific community's opinion are not that relevant.
Kyrgyz Republic—SGBP	Institutions involved are the MoH, Mandatory Health Insurance Fund, Ministry of Finance, national Parliament, and development partners. The Center for Health Policy Analysis contributes with operational research that influences revisions. For instance, a study on sustainability of the SGBP (Manjieva et al. 2007) was used by the Mandatory Health Insurance Fund and development partners to influence the debates on broadening the SGBP. Another example comes from international studies on the importance of folic acid in pregnancy, which were important in including it in the package.
Mexico—Seguro Popular	The FPGC decides the diseases that are of catastrophic nature, then the National Commission for the Social Protection in Health proposes its inclusion and the Technical Committee of the FPGC decides cases and amount. Benefit-inclusion criteria are cost-effectiveness, affordability, financial protection, and the scientific community's opinion.
Nigeria—NHIS-MDG-MCH/MSS/MPHC in Ondo State	The package was designed collaboratively by NHIS, federal MoH, and MoH of the participating states. The criteria for inclusion of benefits are cost-effectiveness, affordability, financial protection, and the scientific community's opinion.
Peru—SIS	The MoH defined the package, with no formal processes for other stakeholders, although it did present the plan to the scientific community and other groups. There are no explicit criteria for revising the package.
Philippines—SP	PhilHealth has a benefits development team and actuarial unit which review the evidence, conduct calculations, and propose benefit package changes to Philhealth's Board. There is no clearly established role for the scientific community or for third-party assessment of evidence. The team conducts cost-effectiveness analysis, however, even though such criteria are not a requirement. Fiscal considerations weigh heavily.
South Africa—ATP	The Care and Support subdirectorate within the HIV, AIDS, and TB Cluster is charged with defining and regularly updating treatment guidelines for management of HIV, AIDS, TB, and STIs, including that for the use of ARVs, and involves consultations with local experts and the MoH. There are two criteria for inclusion of benefits: Affordability (ensured by negotiations with industry) and opinions of the scientific community using international guidelines on drug regimens; and appropriate treatment initiation.
Thailand—UCS	The National Health Security Board (NHSB) is in charge of setting and revising the benefit package. Several stakeholders can nominate topics for evaluation, or potential items for incorporation in the package. Those considered priorities are subject to an HTA conducted by the Health Intervention and Technology Assessment Program (HITAP)—under MoH—or by the Health Systems Research Institute (HSRI)—an autonomous state agency. The results are appraised by a benefit package committee in the NHSB that produces recommendations for the NHSB that makes the final decision. Inclusion/exclusion criteria used are cost-effectiveness, affordability, financial protection, and opinion of the scientific community, although they are not required by law.

table continues next page

TABLE 3.7 *(Continued)*

Country and program	Process and criteria for prioritizing
Tunisia—FMAP	Only MoH is often involved in revising the benefit package. There are no specified criteria for including benefits. However, opinion of the scientific community on treatment protocols is considered by MoH. Only the technical capacities of each facility can limit the package offered, otherwise the patient is referred to a higher-level facility that can provide the services. Poor or nonpoor alike have access to all the benefits provided by a public facility.
Turkey—Green Card	The institutions setting the benefit package are the MoH, Ministry of Finance, Treasury, and the Social Security Institution. The criteria for including benefits are cost-effectiveness, affordability, financial protection, and opinions from the scientific community (scientific community participates particularly for cost-effectiveness studies). The package does not explicitly take into account fiscal impact/budget availability.
Vietnam—SHI	The benefit package was set by MoH, which plays the key role in setting and revising it. Other stakeholders such as the VSS, the Ministry of Finance, and providers are also involved in revisions. There are no processes or criteria formally set for prioritizing and including benefits, and so the package is not usually based on technical criteria. In recent years, for example, the package has been expanded to meet requirements of suppliers that have invested in advanced technology and to keep pace with a fast-growing pharmaceutical market.

Source: UNICO studies.

a similar omission to that seen when the packages were created. Though administrative processes in most countries require initial estimates before policy is changed, they are rarely systematic, and countries frequently revise budgetary allocations in line with requirements. This, of course, carries the risk of the benefit packages being prone to short-term decision-making horizons, often for choices that are politically expedient but not necessarily affordable or sustainable.

Improving Prioritization—Some Views and Approaches

To make informed decisions on prioritizing, some information and evidence require systematic research, as in cost-effectiveness studies or HTAs—though hardly any UNICO countries carried out a systematic HTA save, notably, Thailand (see table 3.7). There may be a case for HTA to be undertaken as a global public good by a shared institution or a set of institutions, with local adaptation mechanisms, as setting up a complete HTA infrastructure and process in each country will duplicate resources and may also be beyond the capacity of many low- and middle-income countries (Glassman et al. 2012).

The Lancet Commission on Global Health in 2035 (Jamison et al. 2013) quotes a study (which became Verguet et al. 2015), in which extended cost-effectiveness analysis was undertaken, tied to preparations for the third edition of *Disease Control Priorities in Developing Countries*.[5] The analysis shows that two interventions having the same effect on reducing mortality can have a different effect on averting poverty, which could then be a criterion for prioritizing interventions to be included in benefit packages. The commission goes on to identify specific essential benefit packages for NCDs, expanding on the WHO benefit package (WHO 2010).

The WHO consultative group on equity and UHC (WHO 2014) suggested that expansion of UHC services should start with cost-effectiveness criteria, and then integrate the concern for vulnerable groups, including financial protection and other criteria. It suggested that the criteria should be designed with wide public participation, ensuring accountability and participatory inputs. The outcome of this process should be explicit criteria that should then guide the country's decisions on prioritizing services.

Among developed countries, in the Netherlands, for instance, the Dunning Committee (Government Committee on Choices in Health Care 1992) helped create filters to determine the basic package of services, using the explicit criteria of medical necessity, efficiency of care, effectiveness of care, and whether the care could be left to the individual. Context-specific considerations swirl around these choices, related to, for instance, equity, quality, utilization, effectiveness, resource availability, and access.

In the United Kingdom, the National Institute for Clinical Excellence has a defined range of £20,000–30,000 per quality-adjusted life year (QALY) to evaluate the cost-effectiveness of new drugs or new technology being assessed for inclusion in the National Health Service (Appleby et al. 2009).

There may be a case for HTA to be undertaken as a global public good by a shared institution or a set of institutions, with local adaptation mechanisms in place, as setting up a complete HTA infrastructure and process in each country implies duplication of resources and may also be far beyond the capacity of many low- and middle-income countries to undertake (Glassman et al. 2012).

Breaking Promises—De Facto Benefit Packages

Despite the increasing focus on explicitly defining the benefit package, the promised package is not in reality available in many UNICO countries. Few UHC programs distinguish between *promised* and *effective* coverage. The explicit benefit packages, positive lists for drugs, and explicit cost-sharing provisions chosen by policy makers aiming to balance cost-effective and necessary medical services with cash-strapped treasuries create explicit rationing by laying out what the coverage allows, and does not. However, the effective provision of promised services is also implicitly rationed.

Despite explicit benefit packages—intended to overcome the challenges of implicit benefit packages—the impaired services reduce the benefit package in reality to only a subset of that promised. Closed-ended payment systems[6] such as capitation (see next section) may also dilute services (Mechanic 1997).

Most beneficiaries enrolled in UNICO programs saw improved access and utilization of health care services compared with the non-covered and nonenrolled populations, but coverage in practice poses implicit rationing. Some examples: Brazilians and Chileans still perceive that quality and access are better in the private sector and are dissatisfied with long waiting times at public providers serving the Sistema Único de Saúde (SUS) and Fonasa programs. In Indonesia, Jamkesmas cardholders are known to prefer paying out of pocket to avoid perceived stigmatization from providers and longer waiting times due to administrative requirements. In the Philippines, the requirement to produce supporting documents for proving eligibility has disproportionately affected poor households, which either do not have such documents or do not know where to get them. In Tunisia, which theoretically has no coverage caps, beneficiaries may be required to buy drugs from private pharmacies, given the shortages at public facilities. Also, shortage of specialists and waiting lists are more generic issues in Tunisia that all users face, not just the members of FMAP.

As a final example, in Vietnam, although the benefit package is theoretically uniform across all membership groups, the variation in capitation rates across subgroups encourages hospitals to underprovide for groups with lower capitation rates, particularly the poor. In addition, bypassing the primary care provider involves a far higher copayment, hitting the poor especially hard and so inducing lower access to referrals and to secondary and tertiary care hospitals. As these hospitals receive a disproportionately large share of government subsidies, this further adds to the pro-rich nature of supply-side subsidies in that country.

Worldwide, exemptions for the poor from cost-sharing provisions are often included in program design, but do not always work as well as they are intended to. These exemptions are vital, as it is increasingly recognized that demand from low-income patients, particularly those with chronic diseases, is highly price sensitive, both for essential and for nonessential care (Schoen et al. 2010). Even absent cost-sharing provisions, the opportunity costs of accessing health care, in view of distance and time involved, can themselves curtail access, particularly for the poorest groups in lower-income countries.

Most health financing programs (not just the UNICO programs) endeavor to align incentives, and thus services that are likely to experience overuse are often subjected to cost-sharing provisions, in contrast to preventive services, which often see exemptions from such provisions or even outright incentives to encourage their use. These exemptions are often offered to the poor and other vulnerable groups to ensure that this is not a serious impediment to their accessing health care services. This is yet another reason to offer incentives for promotional and preventive services that may not experience demand similar to that for curative services. In fact, as cost-sharing provisions constitute OOPE, they are used increasingly with caution.

Among the UNICO programs, cost sharing is rarely required in cost-effective preventive services, such as maternity and public health care services, across all country income groups. It is also not explicitly required in wage-compensation components (wherever offered as part of the benefit package), though such compensation would typically only account for part of the wages that would have otherwise been earned, making such a contribution implicit. However, about one-third of all studied programs require cost sharing for inpatient services and about half require beneficiaries to copay for outpatient services (table 3.8), especially for pharmaceuticals.

Further research will help elucidate the proportion of such cost sharing in the total costs of the covered items, and what proportion of household expenditure is spent on such cost sharing. The equity aspect of cost-sharing provisions, their role in cost containment, and hindrances on access to services all require further exploration.

Studies from OECD countries have shown that cost-sharing provisions for pharmaceutical coverage were nearly universal, while those for primary care outpatient coverage were common but not universal, with Canada, the Netherlands, and the United Kingdom exceptions (Schoen et al. 2010; OECD 2011). Creating positive lists for drugs seemed fairly common across OECD countries (the United Kingdom and United States being notable exceptions where no explicit lists exist) as a cost-containment provision, with the inclusion decisions being increasingly taken by specialized and autonomous entities created by government.

TABLE 3.8
UNICO Programs and Cost-Sharing Provisions, 2012

Country	Cost sharing provisions
Brazil	No
China	Yes
Georgia	No
India—NRHM	Yes
India—RA	No
India—RSBY	No
Indonesia	No
Jamaica	Yes
Kyrgyz Republic	Yes
Massachusetts	Yes
Mexico	No
Nigeria	No
Turkey	Yes
Vietnam	No
Chile	No
Colombia	Yes
Costa Rica	No
Guatemala	No
South Africa	No
Kenya	Yes
Ethiopia	No
Argentina	No
Ghana	No
Philippines	Yes
Tunisia	Yes
Peru	No
Thailand	No

Source: UNICO studies.

These examples demonstrate that the individual program components discussed in this chapter are not only closely linked to the discussions on resources and who is covered, but also those on supply of health care services (chapter 5), and need to be considered holistically.

Contracting Benefits—Engaging Private Providers, Using Closed-Ended Payments, and Improving Linkages to Performance

A whole body of literature demonstrates that the manner in which health care providers are paid can have a significant impact on the costs and quality of their services. The corollary is that payers can design and modify their purchasing and contracting mechanisms to modify provider behavior. Tables 3.9 and 3.10 characterize the provider-payment mechanisms in primary and inpatient settings. Each method has its own

TABLE 3.9
PHC Payment Methods, Characteristics, and Incentives

Payment method	Characteristics	
	Payment based on inputs or outputs?	**Incentives for providers**
Line-item budget	Inputs	Underprovide services; refer to other providers; increase inputs; spend all remaining funds by the end of budget year; no incentive or mechanism to improve efficiency of input mix
Fee for service (fixed-fee schedule and bundling of services)	Outputs	Increase the number of services including above the necessary level; reduce inputs per service
Fee for service (no fixed-fee schedule)	Inputs	Increase number of services; increase inputs
Per capita	Outputs	Improve efficiency of input mix; attract additional enrollees; decrease inputs; underprovide services; refer to other providers; focus on less expensive health promotion and prevention; attempt to select healthier enrollees

Sources: Langenbrunner, Cashin, and O'Dougherty 2009 (adapted from Maceira 1998; Kutzin 2001). Providers paid primarily on inputs have an incentive to maximize inputs and no incentive to increase outputs (or efficiency). This could lead to underproviding services and shifting patients to other levels of care. Systems based on line-item budgets typically face the inefficiency and quality issues that input-based payment mechanisms bring. On the other hand, open-ended fee-for-service (FFS) payments encourage providers to increase the number of services provided. Closed-ended payment systems, such as capitation and case-based payments, in contrast, create incentives for efficiency and to reduce inputs, but may also result in shifting of patients to other levels of care.

TABLE 3.10
Hospital Payment Methods, Characteristics, and Incentives

Payment method	Characteristics			Incentives for providers
	Payment rate set prospectively or retrospectively	Payment to providers made prospectively or retrospectively	Payments based on inputs or outputs	
Line-item budget	Prospectively	Prospectively	Inputs	Underprovide services: refer to other providers; increase inputs; no incentive or mechanism to improve the efficiency of the input mix; incentive to spend all remaining funds by the end of budget year
FFS (fixed-fee schedule and bundling of services	Retrospectively	Retrospectively	Outputs	Increase number of services including above necessary level; reduce inputs per services
FFS (no fixed-fee schedule)	Prospectively	Retrospectively	Inputs	Increase number of services; increase inputs
Per diem	Prospectively	Retrospectively	Outputs	Increase number of days (admission and length of stay); reduce inputs per hospital day; increase bed capacity
Case-based Payments	Prospectively	Retrospectively	Outputs	Increase number of cases, including unnecessary hospitalization; reduce inputs per case; incentive to improve the efficiency of the input mix; reduce length of stay; shift rehabilitation care to the outpatient setting
Global budget	Prospectively	Prospectively	Inputs or Outputs	Underprovide services; refer to other providers; increase inputs; mechanism to improve efficiency of the input mix

Sources: Langenbrunner, Cashin, and O'Dougherty 2009 (adapted from Maceira 1998; Kutzin 2001).

advantages and trade-offs, and its own incentive signals to providers to act in a particular way. In practice, payment methods are increasingly being blended to achieve a more balanced set of signals where the disadvantages of a particular payment method are mitigated by combining it with another.

The UNICO programs found ways to improve delivery of services.[7] To illustrate one such trend, half the programs (13 out of 26) now allow their beneficiaries a choice of using private providers.[8] On the one hand, this indicates an evolution of the stewardship function of the government and its willingness to augment its capacity by engaging the private sector, and on the other it means that program management is increasingly complex and needs adequate contracting and purchasing capacity.

To modernize and innovate their payment systems, many of these programs have introduced performance-based top-ups for public facilities and closed-ended bundled payments for private facilities. Programs in Brazil, Chile, Georgia, Guatemala, Indonesia, the Kyrgyz Republic, Nigeria, the Philippines, Thailand, and Turkey used capitation-based methods, at least in part, to pay their providers for outpatient primary care. The remaining UNICO countries continued using salaries or FFS-based payment systems for outpatient primary care (table 3.11). However, only a subset of these countries used capitation-based payment systems for outpatient specialist care, the rest used FFS.

For inpatient services, UNICO programs have also increasingly adopted case-based payments. These closed-ended, bundled payment systems offer several cost and quality advantages over payment mechanisms like line-item budgets and FFS systems. The UHC programs in Ghana, India, Indonesia, the Kyrgyz Republic, Thailand, Tunisia, and Turkey only use case-based payment methods to compensate inpatient providers. In Chile, Georgia, and Peru, case-based payment methods are used in combination with FFS payment mechanisms. The UCS in Thailand pays for inpatient care by using a blend of DRGs for case-based payments, along with a cap using global budgets, which creates a reinforced cost-containment incentive for providers and keeps costs under control for the treasury.

In OECD countries, while FFS and salary-based payments to physicians still dominate provider-payment methods, several countries have made shifts to closed-ended payments.[9] The switch from line-item budgets to case-based payments and/or global budgets to pay for inpatient care is more widespread, though. Almost all OECD countries that participated in a 2009 OECD survey (OECD 2011) had made this switch, except Spain and Turkey, which continued to use line-item budgets as the main payment mechanism for inpatient services.

Yet these newer provider-payment systems add complexity to designing and running programs, and further underscore the need for greater capacity in supervisory and regulatory agencies. Creating the capacity to set appropriate pricing/reimbursement levels and to undertake contract negotiation and contract management are specialized skills, and need to be created and nurtured in health departments.

TABLE 3.11
Provider-Payment Mechanisms in UNICO Countries, 2011–12

Country	Hospital component (hotel services, nursing care, disposables, tests)	Outpatient primary care contacts	Outpatient specialist contacts	Pharmaceuticals for outpatient services
Argentina		FFS	FFS	
Brazil		CAP + P4P	FFS	None
Chile	FFS or CP	CAP + FFS	FFS	CAP + FFS
China	FFS	FFS	FFS	FFS
Costa Rica		Historical budgets	Historical budgets	Historical budgets
Georgia	FFS/CP	CAP/SAL	FFS/SAL	
Ghana	CP	CP	CP	CP
Guatemala		CAP	CAP	
India—RA	CP	n.a.	n.a.	n.a.
India—RSBY	CP	n.a.	n.a.	n.a.
India—NRHM	SAL	SAL	SAL	SAL
Indonesia	CP	FFS/CAP	FFS	FFS
Jamaica		n/a	n/a	n/a
Kenya		CP	NA	FFS
Kyrgyz Republic	CP	CAP	CAP	RP, CAP
Mexico	SAL—payroll Budgets CP	SAL	SAL	Budgets CP
Nigeria		CAP	CAP	FFS
Peru	CP/FFS	CP/FFS	CP/FFS	CP/FFS
Philippines	FFS	CAP	FFS	None
South Africa	SAL	SAL	SAL	SAL
Thailand	CP	CAP	CAP	CAP
Tunisia	CP	SAL	SAL	FFS
Turkey		CAP, P4P	CAP, P4P	FFS
Vietnam	SAL, FFS, CAP, CP	SAL, FFS, CAP, CP	SAL, FFS, CAP, CP	SAL, FFS, CAP, CP

Source: UNICO studies.
Note: CAP = capitation; CP = case payments; P4P = pay for performance; FFS = fee for service; SAL = salaries; n.a. = not applicable.

Conclusions and Policy Implications

Measuring where a country stands on coverage of health care services (or its benefit package) at a given time against the optimal coverage required for it to qualify as UHC, though crucial for identifying gaps in coverage, poses a much greater challenge than, say, measuring the share of population covered by the same program. There is also the central dilemma in prioritizing a benefit package when multiple objectives tug policy makers in different directions.

Among the UNICO programs, cost sharing is rarely required in cost-effective preventive services, such as maternity and public health care services, across all country income groups, but about one-third require it for inpatient services and about half for outpatient services. Further research is needed to analyze its equity and cost-containment impacts, and any hindrances to access.

Most UNICO countries have yet to take full advantage of priority setting as a necessary, systematic, evidence-based and consultative process. Even if they frequently cited affordability and cost-effectiveness as the most common criteria for initially selecting the content of benefit packages, half had no formal prioritization criteria—nor did most UNICO countries systematically determine affordability. Similarly when revising the package, few conducted in-depth assessments of fiscal impact, expecting to tweak the budget as requirements change.

Nearly all the countries had explicit benefit packages (only three did not) using positive lists or a combination of positive and negative lists. Very few countries, however, used standardized coding systems. Yet despite such apparent openness, many countries' promised package is not in reality always available, presenting a form of implicit rationing.

The UHC programs have, found new ways to contract services, including innovations on payment systems such as performance-based top-ups for public facilities and closed-ended bundled payments for private facilities. Ten programs used capitation-based methods, at least in part, to pay their providers for outpatient primary care. The rest continued using salaries or FFS-based payment systems for outpatient primary care. For inpatient services, UNICO programs have also increasingly adopted case-based payments.

Analysis of the above points to the following implications for policy makers' consideration.

A focus on priority setting using systematic, institutionalized processes and duly considering evidence as well as stakeholder views is a vital and much underused tool in decisions on expanding service coverage. Given that resources will always be limited, policy makers need to choose their goal for health service coverage as well as the sequencing of incremental expansion.

Such decisions often require top-level decisions, especially as increasing amounts of health expenditures are going to drugs and technology, in turn benefiting from delegation to specialized bodies.

NCDs seem to be the widely prevalent gap in service coverage, and need priority attention in view of their overwhelming share of the disease burden. Among UNICO countries, causes of the overall disease burden varied largely by income and region, with some notable exceptions such as Georgia and South Africa. As is true of most countries globally, NCDs were the predominant causes of morbidity and mortality in UNICO countries. At the same time, coverage for NCDs continues to be weak overall across UNICO countries, which also makes NCDs an important focus in many UHC programs.

Delivering promised coverage requires planning and effort. This is crucial because effective benefits in some countries have been cut to a subset of the promised benefit package. Service availability and readiness, and preparing for unforeseen impacts, are as vital as the expansion design itself.

Strengthening the program's management capacity, in particular to contract providers and purchase strategically and well, will be vital areas for capacity building. These needs stem from the increasingly complex world of program management.

Systematic health systems research needs to be strengthened, and will answer many of the knowledge gaps that still exist. Several promising areas for further research touch on the information needed to make decisions on prioritization, including the political economy of choices made for service coverage, assessing how prioritization criteria change, the equity impact of cost sharing (particularly for the most vulnerable) and a full appreciation of cost-effectiveness studies or HTAs. A final area centers on the impact of UNICO UHC programs on broader health systems.

A comprehensive approach to health reform, rather than piecemeal, ad hoc steps that address only a part of the problem, is vital. The fine-grained elements of benefit packages are closely linked not only to discussions on resources and who is covered, but also those on health care providers and the supply of health care services, requiring them to be viewed in a whole-of-system manner.

Notes

1. The International Classification of Diseases (ICD), published by WHO and now in its 10th version (ICD-10), provides a standard system of diagnosis codes to classify disease.
2. Health technology assessment (HTA) is a multidisciplinary process that summarizes information about the medical, social, economic, and ethical issues related to the use of a health technology in a systematic, transparent,

unbiased, robust manner. Its aim is to inform the formulation of safe, effective, health policies that are patient focused and seek to achieve best value. Despite its policy goals, HTA must always be firmly rooted in research and the scientific method. European Network for Health Technology Assessment. "Common Questions. Health Technology Assessment (HTA)." http://www.eunethta.eu/about-us/faq#t287n73. Accessed April 1, 2015.

3. This chapter uses terms employed in the information questionnaire (appendix D). Affordability here refers to the ability of the sponsoring government to prioritize and secure adequate resources for implementing the program, at least in the short term. This is to be contrasted with sustainability, which refers to the medium to long term.

4. The rescue principle makes specific rescue of an individual suffering from a tertiary disease more attractive than invisible public health actions with greater cost-effectiveness or larger benefits. The political economy of benefit packages is often based on what people want to receive, which leads to many benefit packages choosing tertiary cover due to its visibility. The financial protection in the UHC definition intends to cover such services, but sequencing it before other more cost-effective interventions is an issue of political economy.

5. *Disease Control Priorities in Developing Countries* was first published in 1993 as a companion volume to the *World Development Report 1993* focused on investing in health. It included a comprehensive review of the cost-effectiveness of health interventions available for the most common disease conditions affecting the developing world. A second edition was published in 2006 (Jamison et al. 2006) and a third edition is being planned.

6. Closed-ended provider payment mechanisms provide a pre-agreed fee or amount of payment to the providers for a particular set of services (such as all services associated in a single episode of hospitalization), irrespective of the actual inputs and number of services that may need to be provided in a specific case. Thus some part of the risk is shifted to providers and any additional services provided by them for a patient may not result in any additional revenues. In contrast, open-ended provider payment systems allow providers to charge a fee for each service provided, allowing them to receive additional payments by increasing inputs or services.

7. The importance of these advances made in contracting these services, shifting the basis of financing from inputs to outputs, and providing their beneficiaries with a choice of providers is discussed further in chapter 6.

8. Chile, China, Georgia, Ghana, India—RA, India—RSBY, Indonesia, Jamaica, Kenya, the Kyrgyz Republic, Nigeria, the Philippines, and Vietnam.

9. Austria, the Czech Republic, Denmark, Finland, Hungary, Italy, the Netherlands, Norway, Poland, the Slovak Republic, Spain, and the United Kingdom have partially or fully moved to capitation as the payment mechanism for primary care physicians (OECD 2011).

References

Appleby, John, Nancy Devlin, David Parkin, Martin Buxton, and Kalipso Chalkidou. 2009. "Searching for Cost Effectiveness Thresholds in the NHS." *Health Policy* 91: 239–45.

Coen, David, and Mark Thatcher. 2005. "The New Governance of Markets and Non-majoritarian Regulators." *Governance: An International Journal of Policy, Administration, and Institutions* 18 (3): 329–46.

Filmer, Deon, Jeffrey S. Hammer, and Lant H. Pritchett. 2002. "Weak Links in the Chain II: A Prescription for Health Policy in Poor Countries." *The World Bank Research Observer* 17 (1): 47–66.

Flinders, Matthew. 2008. "Delegated Governance and the British State: Walking without Order." Oxford Scholarship Online.

Giedion, Ursula, Ricardo Bitran, and Ignez Tristao, eds. 2014. *Health Benefit Plans in Latin America: A Regional Comparison.* Washington, DC: Social Protection and Health Division, Inter-American Development Bank.

Glassman, Amanda, Kalipso Chalkidou, Ursula K. Giedion, Yot Teerawattananon, Sean Tunis, Jesse B. Bump, and Andres Pichon-Riviere. 2012. "Priority-Setting Institutions in Health Recommendations from a Center for Global Development Working Group." *Global Heart* 7 (1): 13–34.

Government Committee on Choices in Health Care. 1992. *Choices in Health Care.* Rijwsijk, The Netherlands: Ministry of Welfare, Health and Cultural Affairs.

Jamison, Dean T., Joel G. Breman, Anthony R. Measham, George Alleyne, Mariam Claeson, David B. Evans, Prabhat Jha, Anne Mills, and Philip Musgrove, eds. 2006. *Disease Control Priorities in Developing Countries.* Washington, DC: World Bank.

Jamison, Dean T., Lawrence H. Summers, George Alleyne, Kenneth J. Arrow, et al. 2013. "Global Health 2035: A World Converging within a Generation." *The Lancet* 382: 1898–955.

Kutzin, Joseph. 2001. "A Descriptive Framework for Country-Level Analysis of Health Care Financing Arrangements." *Health Policy* 56 (3): 171–204.

———. 2013. "Health Financing for Universal Coverage and Health System Performance: Concepts and Implications for Policy." *Bulletin of the World Health Organization* 91: 602–11.

Landwehr, Claudia, and Katharina Bohm. 2011. "Delegation and Institutional Design in Health-Care Rationing." *Governance: An International Journal of Policy, Administration, and Institutions* 24 (4): 665–88.

Langenbrunner, Jack, Cheryl Cashin, and Sheila O'Dougherty, eds. 2009. *Designing and Implementing Health Care Provider Payment Systems: How-to Manuals.* Washington, DC: World Bank.

Maceira, M. S. 1998. "Provider Payment Mechanisms in Health Care: Incentives, Outcomes and Organizational Impact in Developing Countries." Major Applied Research 2, Working Paper 2, Partnerships for Health Reform Project, Abt Associates Inc., Bethesda, MD.

Manjieva, E., U. Narmanbetov, N. Kadyrova, and M. Jakab. 2007. "Analysis of the Medium-Term Financial Sustainability of the State Guaranteed Benefits Package." Policy Research Paper 43, World Health Organization and Health Policy Analysis Center, Bishkek.

Mechanic, David. 1997. "Muddling through Elegantly: Finding the Proper Balance in Rationing Explicit Rationing at the Clinical Level Is Likely to Cause More Harm than Good." *Health Affairs* 16 (5): 83–92.

Murray, Christopher J. L., Theo Vos, Rafael Lozano, Mohsen Naghavi, Abraham D. Flaxman, Catherine Michaud, Majid Ezzati, et al. 2013. "Disability-Adjusted Life Years (DALYs) for 291 Diseases and Injuries in 21 Regions, 1990–2010: A Systematic Analysis for the Global Burden of Disease Study 2010." *The Lancet* 380 (9859): 2197–223.

OECD (Organisation for Economic Co-operation and Development). 2011. "Burden of Out-of-Pocket Health Expenditure." Health at a Glance, OECD Indicators.

Paris, V., M. Devaux, and L. Wei. 2010. "Health Systems Institutional Characteristics: A Survey of 29 OECD Countries." OECD Health Working Papers, 50. OECD Publishing, Paris. http://dx.doi.org/10 .1787/5kmfxfq9qbnr-en.

Schoen, Cathy, Robin Osborn, David Squires, Michelle M. Doty, Roz Pierson, and Sandra Applebaum. 2010. "How Health Insurance Design Affects Access to Care and Costs, by Income, in Eleven Countries." *Health Affairs* 29 (12): 2323–334.

Verguet, Stéphane, Ramanan Laxminarayan, and Dean T. Jamison. 2015. "Universal Public Finance of Tuberculosis Treatment in India: An Extended Cost-Effectiveness Analysis." *Health Economics* 24 (3): 318–32.

WHO (World Health Organization). 2010. *The World Health Report—Health Systems Financing: The Path to Universal Coverage*. Geneva: WHO.

———. 2014. "Making Fair Choices in the Path to Universal Health Coverage." Final report of the WHO Consultative Group on Equity and Universal Health Coverage, Members of the WHO Consultative Group, Geneva.

WHO and IBRD (International Bank for Reconstruction and Development)/ World Bank. 2014. "Monitoring Progress towards Universal Health Coverage at Country and Global Levels: Framework, Measures and Targets." WHO and the World Bank Group, Geneva.

Wong, Holly, and Ricardo Bitran. 1999. "Module 5 Designing a Benefits Package." Prepared for the Flagship Course on Health Sector Reform and Sustainable Financing, World Bank Institute.

CHAPTER 4

Managing Money: Financing the Bottom-Up Expansion of Universal Health Coverage

This chapter identifies key trends, highlights good practices where evident, and summarizes policy implications for financing universal health coverage (UHC) expansion in the 24 Universal Health Coverage Studies Series (UNICO) countries. It focuses on two aspects of the UHC cube (chapter 1) that are relevant from the perspective of UHC program financing: the *height* of the cube, representing the extent of financial protection from direct costs accorded by UHC programs at the time and point of seeking care; and the *volume* of the inner cube, representing the extent of pooled financing (a function of all three dimensions of the cube: number of people covered, services covered, and extent of financial coverage provided by UHC programs).

Adequate resources for expanding UHC programs are typically a prominent policy consideration across developing countries. Resource needs are in large part dependent on country context, the extent of population coverage of the UHC program, risk profile of beneficiaries and their utilization rates, costs of inputs, nature and extent of benefits provided, and how the health system is organized and financed. Resource availability depends on the willingness and ability of beneficiaries to contribute, administrative capacity of countries to collect contributions, fiscal capacity of governments to subsidize coverage for those who cannot contribute, and extent of cross-subsidization possibilities from richer to poorer beneficiaries.

Health financing, however, is not just about resource adequacy: it is also about the efficiency, equity, and effectiveness of the ways in which resources are raised, pooled, allocated, and used to achieve desired health system outcomes, such as those for UHC (Hsiao 2007). Health financing strategies may also require assessments related to financial sustainability and the impact of reforms on the broader economy. UHC-related health financing reforms can potentially improve health outcomes, mitigate household vulnerability, and reduce the risk of impoverishment from catastrophic health spending.

They can also, though, have unintended consequences: policies to improve revenue collection may result in increased labor costs, encouraging informality as well as raising the fiscal burden on governments (Wagstaff 2010), while rising health care costs, unless mitigated by strategic purchasing and efficiency gains, can threaten the financial sustainability of health care reforms.

Health financing is a core function—one of six fundamental health system "building blocks" in World Health Organization's (WHO's) conceptual framework—that normally includes an assessment of three subareas: revenue collection; risk pooling and resource allocation; and purchasing (Gottret and Schieber 2006; WHO 2010). This chapter uses this simple health financing framework to assess the modalities of revenue generation, risk pooling, and resource allocation policy choices that financed the expansion of UHC programs across UNICO countries.[1] It does so to tackle several key issues: How much did the expansion in coverage cost? Did expenditures vary systematically by country income, extent of population coverage, benefit package coverage, and by the degree of financial protection accorded by UHC programs? To what extent were UHC program expenditures complemented by other sources of health financing? What are some prominent sources and contribution mechanisms for financing UHC programs? What kinds of cost-sharing modalities were evident across UHC programs? And what were some of the policy choices made with regard to risk pooling and resource allocation methods implemented across UNICO countries?

For ease of context, health financing information is categorized across the five broad subcategories of UHC programs introduced in earlier chapters, the first on the supply side, the last four on the demand side (and see table 1.2):

- supply-side programs (SSPs): these focused primarily on improving service provision via bolstering supply-side investments, and were generally open to all population subgroups;

- poor and vulnerable programs (PVPs): these represented demand-side programs financed by general taxes that paid providers for services provided exclusively to poor and vulnerable population subgroups;

- informal sector programs (ISPs): these provided coverage to all those not covered by formal sector coverage programs, including the non-poor informal sector;

- social health insurance programs (SHI+): these provided the poor and vulnerable with tax-financed coverage within national single-program UHC initiatives that included contributory enrollment of the formal sector and voluntary enrollment for the nonpoor informal sector; and

- social health insurance programs with de facto mandatory enrollment for the nonpoor informal sector (SHI++).

In four subsections the rest of the chapter explores some of the issues of financing UHC programs—levels of financing; sources and contribution methods; cost-sharing modalities; and risk pooling and resource allocation—before summarizing general health financing trends across the 26 UNICO programs and highlighting good practices and key policy implications.

Spending Some, Leveraging More

The median annual UHC program expenditure per beneficiary in 2011 across the 26 UNICO programs was US$39, about 1.4 percent of gross domestic product (GDP) per capita (table 4.1). UHC program expenditures per beneficiary varied more than 100-fold across the 24 countries: such annual expenditures exceeded US$500 in South Africa and Costa Rica, but fell short of US$5 in Kenya, Nigeria, Ethiopia, and India. In South Africa and Costa Rica, expenditures averaged around 7 percent of per capita GDP on their UHC programs, in Kenya and Nigeria only 0.04 percent and 0.1 percent.

UHC program expenditures per beneficiary were strongly correlated with per capita GDP (figure 4.1). This partly reflects differences in benefits provided and in the supply- versus demand-side modality: some of the lowest expenditures were among SSPs that provided primary care (such as Ethiopia, Kenya, and India) or those that focused on maternal and child health (MCH) benefits (Nigeria, for example). Another factor is that input costs, especially for health-related nontradable goods and services, tend to be low in lower-income countries (Murray and Tandon 2008). Still, as evident in some of the statistics on health outcomes and coverage rates summarized in appendix B, lower expenditures are also likely indicative of the generally shallower depth and poorer quality of coverage accorded both by UHC programs and by health systems in lower-income countries.

Expenditures for UHC programs across most UNICO countries were also generally low as a share of GDP: the median UHC program expenditure share of GDP was only about 0.4 percent.[2] In 18 of 24 UNICO countries, UHC program expenditures were less than 1 percent of GDP (figure 4.2). In five additional countries—Brazil, Colombia, Thailand, the Kyrgyz Republic, and Chile—UHC program expenditures were

TABLE 4.1
Annual UHC Program Expenditures in UNICO Countries, 2011

| Country | UHC program | UHC program typology | UHC program expenditure per beneficiary | |
			US$	Share of GDP per capita (%)
Kenya	Health Sector Services Fund	SSP	0.3	0.04
Nigeria	National Health Insurance Scheme	SSP	2	0.1
Ethiopia	Health Extension Program	SSP	5	1.5
India	National Rural Health Mission	SSP	4	0.3
	Rashtriya Swasthya Bima Yojna	PVP	2	0.1
	Rajiv Aarogyasri	PVP	3	0.2
Guatemala	Expansion of Coverage Program	SSP	7	0.2
Indonesia	Jamkesmas	PVP	7	0.2
Philippines	National Health Insurance Fund	SHI+	11	0.5
Peru	Seguro Integral de Salud	PVP	16	0.3
Kyrgyz Republic	Mandatory Health Insurance Fund	SHI+	26	2.3
Vietnam	Social Health Insurance	SHI+	26	1.7
China	National Rural Cooperative Medical Scheme	ISP	38	0.7
Ghana	National Health Insurance Scheme	SHI+	39	2.4
Argentina	Plan Nacer	ISP	42	0.4
Tunisia	Free Medical Assistance for the Poor	PVP	63	1.4
Thailand	Universal Coverage Scheme	ISP	78	1.5
Georgia	Medical Insurance Program	PVP	99	3.1
Jamaica	Jamaica National Health Fund	SSP	108	2.0
Colombia	Subsidized Regime	ISP	120	1.7
Mexico	Seguro Popular	ISP	122	1.3
Brazil	Family Health Strategy	SSP	125	1.0
Turkey	Green Card	PVP	209	2.0
Chile	Fonasa	SHI++	313	2.2
South Africa	Antiretroviral Treatment Program	SSP	556	7.0
Costa Rica	Caja Costarricense de Seguridad Social	SHI++	589	6.8
Median			39	1.4

Source: UNICO studies.

FIGURE 4.1

UHC Program Expenditures per Beneficiary versus GDP per Capita in UNICO Countries, 2011

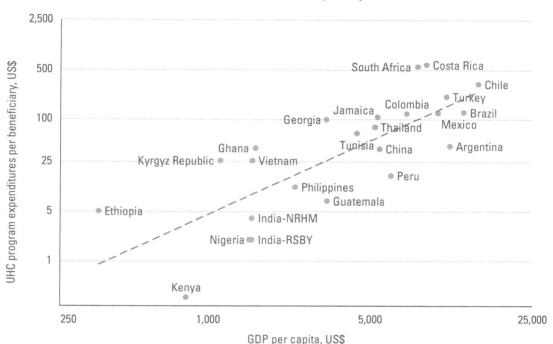

Sources: UNICO studies; World Development Indicators database.
Note: Y-axis and x-axis log scale.

roughly 1–2 percent of GDP. Variations in the expenditure share of GDP reflect differences across at least three key UHC program dimensions, namely the proportion of the national population covered by the UHC program; the limited versus comprehensive nature of services covered; and the extent to which UHC program financing was complemented by other forms of financing (for example, by supply-side financing in demand-side financed UHC programs).

The two countries with the highest UHC program expenditure share of GDP (Costa Rica and Chile) provided comprehensive coverage as part of SHI++ UHC programs to relatively large shares of their respective national populations. Among these, Costa Rica was a clear outlier with UHC program expenditures at 6.2 percent of GDP, about three times as high as Chile. Costa Rica's program covered a larger share of its population: 91 percent compared with 78 percent in Chile.[3] Costa Rica is also unique in that providers are owned and managed by the country's social insurance program and not by the government. Costa Rica spent a larger share of its government budget on health than Chile; Costa Rica also had lower out-of-pocket expenditure (OOPE) as a share of total health expenditures than Chile (table 4.2).

FIGURE 4.2
UHC Program Expenditures as Share of GDP in UNICO Countries, 2011

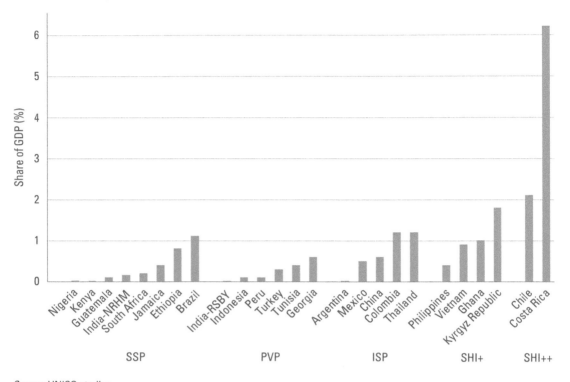

Source: UNICO studies.

TABLE 4.2
Key Health Financing Indicators for SHI++ Programs, 2011

	Costa Rica	Chile
GDP per capita (US$)	8,661	14,513
UHC program population coverage (%)	91.0	78.0
UHC program expenditure share of GDP (%)	6.2	2.1
UHC program expenditure share of public health expenditure (%)	81.0	57.0
Public health expenditure share of GDP (%)	7.6	3.4
Public health expenditure share of government budget (%)	28.0	14.8
OOPE share of total health expenditures (%)	23.0	33.0

Sources: UNICO studies; World Development Indicators database.

The Kyrgyz Republic had the third-highest UHC program spending share of GDP (1.8 percent), covering 76 percent of the population; Thailand and Colombia's were the fourth and fifth highest. Thailand's UHC program provided coverage to an estimated 71 percent of the population, accounting for 40 percent of all public spending on health in the country; Colombia— with 47 percent coverage and UHC program expenditures at 24 percent of total public spending on health—rounded out the top five countries.

At 1.1 percent and 0.8 percent of GDP, respectively, UHC programs in Brazil and Ethiopia were the only two SSPs in the top 10 countries in terms of UHC program expenditures that provided noncomprehensive limited coverage (for primary care only) but for relatively large shares (more than two-thirds) of their populations. Two of the UHC programs with the lowest expenditure shares of GDP—Nigeria and Argentina— provided limited MCH-related coverage to less than 5 percent of their populations. Expenditures for SHI+/SHI++ UHC programs, on average, represented a higher share of GDP and of total public expenditure on health than UHC programs that either provided disease or level-specific coverage or those that provided coverage for poor-specific population subgroups as part of separate, targeted programs (table 4.3). However, the per beneficiary expenditures under SHI+ and SHI++ programs were not always the same for contributory and noncontributory populations. In some countries such as Vietnam, expenditures for noncontributory members (sometimes by design, location, responsiveness, or other factors) were lower than for contributory members.

TABLE 4.3
UHC Program Expenditures by Program Typology, 2011

UHC program typology	Program	Total UHC program expenditure (%)	
		Share of GDP	Share of public health expenditures
SSP	Brazil, Ethiopia, Guatemala, India—NRHM, Jamaica, Kenya, Nigeria, South Africa	0.3	8.3
PVP	Georgia, India—RSBY, India—RA, Indonesia, Peru, Tunisia, Turkey	0.3	11.3
ISP	Argentina, China, Colombia, Mexico, Thailand	0.7	20.9
SHI+	Ghana, Kyrgyz Republic, Philippines, Vietnam	1.0	36.0
SHI++	Chile, Costa Rica	4.2	68.7

Source: UNICO studies.

A key point is that, in almost all UNICO countries, UHC program expenditures are marginal: they do not represent the full cost of care, which can be seen also in spending comparisons: UHC program expenditure share in total public health expenditures, and per beneficiary UHC program expenditures as a share of per capita public health expenditures. The median UHC program expenditure share in total public spending on health was about 14 percent (figure 4.3). Costa Rica and Chile aside, UHC program expenditures were generally less than 50 percent of total public spending on health in UNICO countries. In some countries this would be expected as the UHC program did not provide comprehensive coverage, but even some UHC programs that did provide such coverage did not cover the full costs of the benefit package.

Kenya, for example, had one of the lowest expenditures (around US$0.30; 0.02 percent of GDP; and 0.9 percent of public expenditure on health) among all UHC programs. This was partly because the program was designed to finance only operating and other incremental costs for facilities to provide primary care services included in the Kenya Essential Package of Health Care Services. Similarly, Peru's UHC program was

FIGURE 4.3
UHC Program Expenditure Share in Total Public Health Expenditures in UNICO Countries, 2011

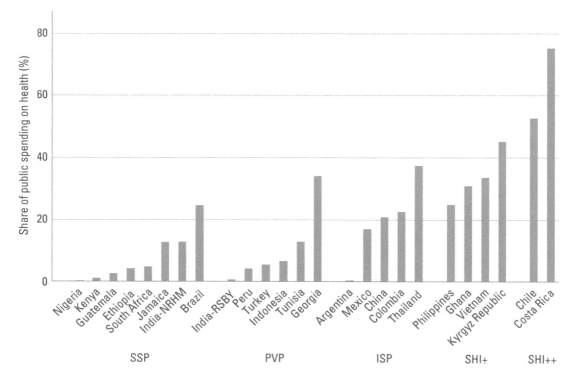

Sources: UNICO studies; World Development Indicators database.

designed to cover only direct user fees at public facilities, with financing calculated only to cover variable costs of inputs, Tunisia's covered only user fee payments for its beneficiaries, and Argentina's only the incremental costs of providing coverage.

In other UHC programs, the partial coverage of costs was implicit: at US$7 per beneficiary per year (0.1 percent of GDP), Indonesia's UHC program covered a small proportion of costs (expenditures by other SHI programs, in contrast, were four to five times as high) with government supply-side expenditures cofinancing provision of care at public facilities. (For example, salaries of health workers at public facilities were paid out of government coffers separately.) Similar arrangements were evident to varying degrees in the Philippines, Thailand, and Vietnam. In almost all UNICO countries that provided comprehensive coverage, UHC program expenditures per beneficiary were lower than per capita public expenditures on health, sometimes hugely so, suggesting cross-subsidization by supply-side and other public spending on health. Georgia and South Africa were exceptions (figure 4.4). In South Africa, this was likely a

FIGURE 4.4

UHC per Beneficiary Program Expenditures as a Share of per Capita Public Health Expenditures in UNICO Countries, 2011

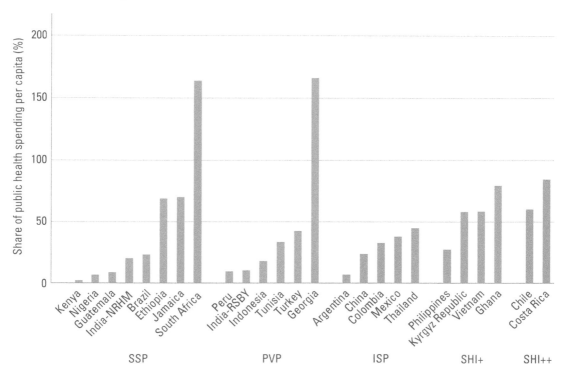

Source: UNICO studies; World Development Indicators database.

result of the relatively high cost of HIV/AIDS-related coverage. In Georgia, the UHC program contracted private insurers who then contracted care from private providers, likely necessitating full-cost coverage.

UNICO countries spanned a wide range on public health expenditures as a share of GDP. About half of them spent more than expected (with Costa Rica a clear outlier) and the other half less than expected relative to their income (with Indonesia the lowest spender) (figure 4.5).

UNICO countries expanded coverage during a period of conducive macroeconomic conditions. They showed faster GDP growth than non-UNICO developing countries over 2000–12, and with few exceptions had a government deficit of less than 3 percent of GDP and government debt of below 60 percent of GDP (appendix B). Apart from Kenya and Ethiopia, UNICO countries increased their public health expenditure as a share in GDP over 2000–12, reflected in a rise in the share of health in public expenditure (figure 4.6). UNICO countries prioritized health more than non-UNICO countries: health was 12.5 percent of the overall government budget versus 10.3 percent in non-UNICO countries in 2011.[4]

FIGURE 4.5
Public Expenditure Share of GDP versus GDP per Capita, 2011 (UNICO Countries Highlighted)

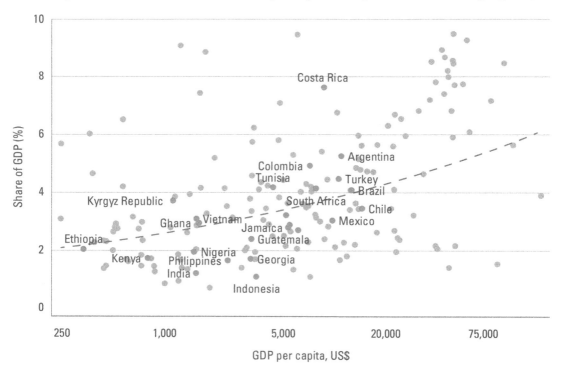

Source: World Development Indicators database.
Note: X-axis logged.

FIGURE 4.6

Annual Growth in Public Health Expenditure as Shares of Public Expenditure and of GDP, 2000–12 (UNICO Countries Highlighted)

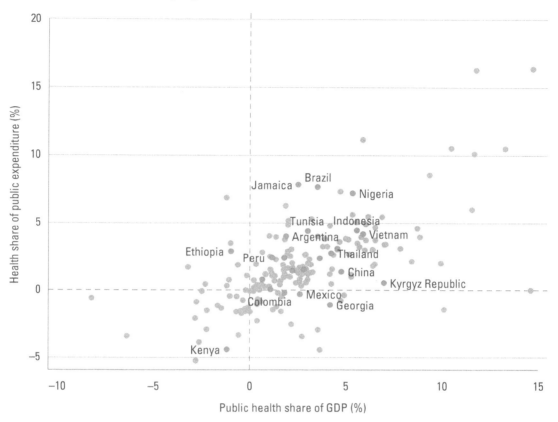

Source: World Development Indicators database.

While most UNICO countries increased the public health expenditure share of GDP, by the end of this period the median was the same among UNICO and non-UNICO developing countries (both were roughly 3 percent of GDP), less than half the median for high-income countries (7.1 percent). This suggests that in terms of financing, the expansion in coverage in UNICO countries represented more of a "catching-up" of public expenditures on health with other developing countries that were spending more on health in 2000. This catching-up was facilitated by generally faster rates of economic growth and conducive macroeconomic conditions.

There were no consistent trends in methods used to estimate and derive costs of UHC programs. Costing health programs can have many potential advantages: it focuses attention on making benefits more explicit and on what exactly needs to be financed to realize UHC, potentially reducing systemic moves toward implicit rationing (if realized allocations reflect costs); it can serve as a powerful signal to those charged with allocating resources, such as ministries of finance, on the type and size of commitments needed to deliver services; and it can be a guide to helping anchor purchaser–provider financing relationships, helping identify and address potential sources of inefficiencies. In reality, however, these advantages were often subsumed by the exigencies of budget constraints, and there is little evidence from UNICO that costing made an appreciable difference to decisions on resource allocation. (Similar conclusions are noted in Kutzin, Cashin, and Jakab 2010.) Another costing challenge is that resources go to health facilities, and are not directly linked to the benefits or services provided.

In many UNICO countries, final UHC program resource allocations were a result of a combination of historical budgets, benchmarking, best guesswork, and back-and-forth negotiations between stakeholders, with only part of the allocation decision reportedly informed by detailed costing exercises. Only a minority of UHC programs stated that they used actuarial analysis (box 4.1) to derive estimates, including Argentina, Costa Rica, Georgia, the Kyrgyz Republic, Mexico, the Philippines, South Africa, Thailand, and Turkey. It was unclear whether costing, the type of costing methodology (such as actuarial analysis or other forms), and the scope of what was costed (average or marginal costs) had any impact on UHC program allocations. Nor was it clear whether, or to what extent, the estimates from the costing exercises in the minority fed through into those countries' final allocations.

To summarize, the levels of UHC program expenditure varied widely across UNICO countries—in part determined by the extent of population coverage, benefits provided, and UHC program typology—and were strongly correlated with national income. Most countries channeled UHC program expenditures from the demand side, complementing traditional supply-side financing of the public health system. UHC spending did not generally appear excessive relative to GDP, as a share of public spending, or as a share of public spending on health.

The implications of the relative size and channeling modalities of resources is that UHC programs are serving as a small but potentially strategic and crucial part of the overall resource envelope needed to provide coverage. UHC programs are covering flexible operating costs and incentives, reflecting financing at the margin, not the average, but nevertheless potentially serving as a powerful tool to make providers and beneficiaries change behavior so as to help attain desired health system outcomes.[5]

BOX 4.1
What Is Actuarial Analysis?

Actuarial analysis is a form of statistical analysis, typically conducted using health-related financial cost data when calculating insurance premium rates or otherwise determining expenditure needs. Actuarial analysis entails estimation of average expenditures of a risk pool so that financing needs can be estimated to ensure that revenues balance expected outlays. Actuarial models often exploit historical claims and utilization data—combined with adjustments made to account for population and inflationary trends—to project expected expenditures. Financial sustainability, or "actuarial soundness," implies that expected expenditures (including administrative costs and any reserve requirements) for a risk pool be less than or equal to expected revenues.

Traditional costing methods—for example, top-down costing (which estimates and allocates aggregate outlays across activities) and bottom-up costing (which costs granular service delivery activities and aggregates them up to estimate outlays)—generally focus on a production approach to estimating resource outlays that may be needed to deliver health care services, taking the consumption of health care services largely as a given. Actuarial analysis, in contrast, takes the production of health care services largely as a given, focusing instead on estimating costs from a consumption approach, probabilistically determining utilization and associated expected expenditures that would be needed to finance health care from a pool of financial resources.

Sources: Cichon et al. 1999; Wang et al. 2012.

Collecting Contributions—Government and Other Sources

Revenue collection is the process by which health systems obtain funds from households, workers, domestic organizations (including governments and firms), and external donors (WHO 2000). Countries can use a range of sources to collect revenues: general government revenues, mandatory SHI contributions (usually salary-based payroll contributions from individuals and employers), voluntary insurance contributions, donations (domestic and external sources), health savings accounts, and direct OOPE (WHO 2000). Apart from adequacy, key considerations include the efficiency and equity impact of the modalities for raising funds, feasibility, political support from key stakeholders, cost versus benefits, and administrative capacity (McIntyre 2007).

Coverage for the poor across all UNICO countries was always noncontributory, whether or not they were covered under separate targeted programs or as part of SHI+/SHI++ UHC programs, with exemptions from direct payments at point and time of service. Coverage for the poor was financed by governments, external sources, or earmarked contributions from parallel formal sector risk pools. Under SHI+/SHI++ programs (see table 4.3), there was also some cross-subsidization by contributory members. Table 4.4 summarizes the revenue sources across UNICO UHC programs.

Government and External Financing

Government revenues were the dominant source of financing across all the programs. In 14 of the 24 countries, UHC programs were entirely financed by a combination of revenues from the central government, subnational governments, or external sources (see table 4.4). UHC programs in Georgia, Indonesia, Peru, Thailand, and Turkey were almost entirely financed by central government revenues. UHC programs in Brazil, India, Mexico, and Nigeria were financed by a combination of central and subnational government revenues (in part reflecting fiscal decentralization in these countries).[6]

Five UHC programs (in Argentina, Ethiopia, Guatemala, Kenya, and South Africa) were financed by a combination of central government and external funds. In Guatemala, external financing accounted for 28 percent of UHC program revenues. About half the financing for South Africa's UHC program came from the U.S. PEPFAR program.

Even though not prominent in the direct financing of most UHC program programs, National Health Accounts data indicate that external sources make up more than 5 percent of total health spending in several UNICO countries, notably lower-income countries such as Ethiopia, Kenya, Ghana, the Kyrgyz Republic, Nigeria, and Georgia. In Ethiopia and Kenya—two of the three low-income UNICO countries—external sources accounted for more than 15 percent of total health spending. In these countries, external sources were likely financing UHC program programs indirectly, via general budget support or financing of complementary programs that often provide resources for general health system inputs (or a mix of both).

Most UNICO countries use earmarking for financing some proportion of government-financed UHC program revenues (box 4.2). One form of earmarking for UHC programs—mandatory social insurance contributions—was significant in Costa Rica (95 percent of total UHC program financing), the Philippines (75 percent), and, to a lesser extent, Chile (39 percent), Vietnam (34 percent), Ghana (15 percent), and the Kyrgyz Republic (15 percent). In all six countries, UHC programs are embedded in SHI+/SHI++ comprehensive UHC programs that pooled

TABLE 4.4

Revenue Collection Sources and Contribution Mechanisms across UNICO UHC Programs, 2011

Country	Government			External	Beneficiaries			Other	Total
	Central	Subnational	Total government		Mandatory premium	Voluntary premium	Point of service		
Argentina		24	24	76[a]					100
Brazil	26	74	100						100
Chile	61		61		39[b]				100
China	45	39	84			16			100
Colombia	47	11	58					42[c]	100
Costa Rica	5		5		95[d]				100
Ethiopia	70		70	30					100
Georgia	100		100						100
Ghana	61		61	2	15	4		18[e]	100
Guatemala	72		72	28					100
India[f]	85	15[g]	100						100
Indonesia	100		100						100
Jamaica	59		59					41[h]	100
Kenya	25		25	75					100
Kyrgyz Republic	68	11	79		15[i]		6		100
Mexico[j]	74	26	100						100
Nigeria	77	23	100						100
Peru	99		99				1[k]		100
Philippines	7	7	14		75	11			100
South Africa	50		50	50[l]					100
Thailand	100		100						100
Tunisia	70		70				10[m]	20[n]	100

table continues next page

TABLE 4.4 *(Continued)*

Country	Government			External	Beneficiaries			Other	Total
	Central	Subnational	Total government		Mandatory premium	Voluntary premium	Point of service		
Turkey	100		100						100
Vietnam	10	30	40		34	18		9[o]	100
Average	58	11	70	11	10	1	1	7	100

Source: UNICO studies.
a. World Bank financing channeled via central government.
b. Information on separation of contributions from mandatory versus voluntary enrollments was unavailable.
c. Cross-subsidization from parallel risk pool (Contributory Regime) that covers the formal sector and in which 1.5% of payroll tax is earmarked as contributions to the UHC program (Subsidized Regime); Cabrera 2011.
d. Information on separation of contributions from mandatory versus voluntary enrollments not available.
e. Interest payments on reserves and other sources of income.
f. Numbers reported in tables are for NRHM; RSBY is 75–25% financed by central-state governments; and RA is entirely financed by the Andhra Pradesh state government.
g. This represents the maximum amount that the states are expected to contribute; in reality, several states have not contributed this amount.
h. Earmarked payroll levy on parallel National Insurance Scheme.
i. Includes voluntary enrollment contributions.
j. In principle, Mexico's UHC program is also supposed to be financed by contributions from nonpoor enrollees, although in practice very few (<1%) of enrolled households contribute to it.
k. Registration fees.
l. PEPFAR.
m. Copayments are charged only from near-poor enrollees who pay a subsidized tariff.
n. Financing from parallel risk pool covering the formal sector.
o. Subsidized payments by the social insurance program in order to cover pensioners.

contributions from formal sector populations with government-subsidized premium payments for the poor.

Half the UHC programs also used other forms of earmarking, most prominently in Ghana where a 2.5 percent value-added tax (VAT) levy was earmarked for UHC program financing, accounting for almost half UHC program financing in that country. In Costa Rica, the premiums for noncontributory members were financed by the central government partly out of taxes on luxury goods, liquor, beer, soda, and other imported goods. About 25 percent of contributions for India's RA program came from earmarked taxes on alcohol.[7] About 41 percent of contributions for Jamaica's National Health Fund, which covers NCD-related benefits, came from earmarked payroll taxes of 0.5 percent on earnings up to JMD$500,000, paid by both employers and employees in a parallel formal sector risk pool (the National Insurance Scheme), and the rest from earmarked tobacco taxes and special consumption taxes on alcohol,

---

BOX 4.2
Earmarking

Earmarking—also referred to as dedicated, hypothecated, ring-fenced, or tagged taxation—typically refers to "... the practice of designating or dedicating specific revenues to the financing of specific public services" (Buchanan 1963). McLeary (1991) distinguishes three forms to categorize sources of government-mandated financing: a *specific* earmarked tax for a *specific* end-use, for example, mandatory SHI premiums; a *specific* earmarked tax for *general* end use, such as earmarked taxes for financing government health expenditures more generally; and a *general* tax earmarked for a *specific* end use, such as a fixed percentage of government revenues or expenditures earmarked for health spending.

Earmarking is a contentious issue. Some macroeconomists view it as an imposition of an unnecessary constraint on fiscal policy making, reducing macroeconomic policy flexibility and hindering allocative efficiency. Theoretically, earmarking may be justified on the basis of the benefit principle in that those who are taxed directly get the benefits from the revenues raised. Earmarking may also be favored if there is clear evidence of willingness to pay additional taxes if they are to be used for a well-defined purpose. Proponents argue that earmarking can potentially protect certain forms of spending from political and macroeconomic vicissitudes: for instance, if health spending is low or unstable, they argue that earmarking is a way to insulate health spending from other competing publicly funded activities, or signals increasing government prioritization of the sector.

Strict earmarking may, however, lead to over- or underfunding of targeted activities and there are numerous examples where earmarked funds have been diverted to other activities, especially in poor governance settings. Earmarking some sources of revenue may also be ineffective in raising additional resources: for instance, mandating contributory enrollment from those who are nonpoor in the informal sector is unlikely to raise much revenue in countries with large levels of informality, given enforcement and adverse-selection problems.

One area where earmarking is potentially effective is in taxing consumption of tobacco, alcohol, and other unhealthy products. Fiscal policy can serve as a powerful tool for inducing desirable health-improving behavioral responses, while raising revenues that could be channeled to finance government health spending—a form of risk-adjusted premium payments, as it were.

Sources: Buchanan 1963; McLeary 1991; Schiavo-Campo 2007; Prakongsai, Patcharanarumol, and Tangcharoensathien 2008; ADB 2012.

---

petroleum, and motor vehicles. Colombia's UHC program was financed in part out of payroll contributions but not from enrollees; instead, there was a "solidarity" cross-subsidized contribution from a parallel risk pool covering the formal sector (Tunisia used a similar mechanism).

Most countries have adopted weak forms of earmarking, augmenting revenues from earmarked sources with general revenue financing. Some earmarked funds for health spending, but not specifically for UHC programs (table 4.5). Guatemala, for example, earmarked taxes but

TABLE 4.5
Earmarked Taxes as a Source of Government Health Revenue

Type of earmarking	Country	Description
Specific taxes earmarked for financing UHC programs	Colombia	Earmarked payroll tax from parallel formal sector insurance program
	Costa Rica	Taxes on luxury goods, liquor, beer, soda, and other imported goods to finance noncontributory regime
	India	Earmarked taxes on alcohol for RA
	Jamaica	Earmarked taxes on tobacco, alcohol, petroleum, and motor vehicles; earmarked payroll tax in parallel formal sector insurance program
	Tunisia	Earmarked transfers from parallel formal sector insurance program
Specific taxes earmarked for financing general government health spending (or for financing other non-UHC program health programs)	Chile	Tobacco taxes, customs revenues, and sales of shares in public health enterprises earmarked for financing SHI reform (AUGE)
	Colombia	Earmarked state-level taxes on tobacco and alcohol for financing general government health spending
	Guatemala	Earmarked alcohol and tobacco taxes for financing general government health spending
	Mexico	Earmarked alcohol and tobacco taxes for financing general government health spending
	Thailand	Earmarked alcohol and tobacco taxes to support the Thailand Health Promotion Fund
General taxes earmarked for financing UHC programs, other non-UHC program health programs, or general government health spending	Chile	Earmarked 1% VAT for AUGE
	Ghana	Earmarked 2.5% VAT
	Brazil	Federal health spending equal to health spending in previous year adjusted for changes in nominal GDP; minimum 12% of state expenditure and 15% of municipal expenditure earmarked for health
	Vietnam	Increase in government spending on health has to be higher than increase in overall government spending by law (Resolution No. 18/2008/NQ-QH12 in 2008)

Sources: UNICO studies; for Vietnam general taxes: Grover 2011.
Note: The taxes are other than mandatory SHI premiums.

the revenues went to the general health budget and not just the UHC program. Similarly, earmarking for health cannot be traced specifically to the UHC program in Brazil even though 6–7 percent of federal revenues, 12 percent of state revenues, and 15 percent of municipal revenues are constitutionally mandated for health. In Chile, the government passed a law to raise VAT from 18 percent to 19 percent, and the incremental VAT revenues are used to finance the country's AUGE reform, introduced in 2005. Colombia earmarks taxes on alcohol and tobacco for financing health, including some interventions provided to UHC program enrollees.

A proportion of sin taxation on tobacco and alcohol consumption is earmarked to support the Thailand Health Promotion Fund, an independent body that supports health promotion activities, including improving health awareness and behavioral change. Public health spending is protected by law in Vietnam: the National Assembly passed Resolution No. 18/2008/NQ-QH12 in 2008 to protect and promote government spending on health; according to Article 2 of the resolution, the government would commit "… to increase the share of annual state budget allocations for health, and to ensure that the growth rate of spending on health is greater than the growth rate of overall spending through the state budget" (Grover 2011).

Earmarking was possibly linked to prioritization: health's share of the government budget in UNICO countries that earmarked was 14 percent, higher than among those UNICO countries that did not earmark (11 percent) and among non-UNICO developing countries (11 percent). In Vietnam, for instance, annual growth in government health allocations generally exceeded average growth of the total government budget (Van Tien et al. 2011).

Voluntary Contributions

Voluntary contributions are not a significant source of financing for UHC programs in UNICO countries. In most of these countries, formal sector workers make mandatory contributions to a social health insurance program and UHC policies include tax financing for the poor and vulnerable. Policies encouraging voluntary contributions are mostly directed to nonpoor informal sector workers.

UNICO countries that allow or encourage voluntary contributory enrollment of nonpoor informal sector beneficiaries include most of the countries with UHC programs targeting the poor and vulnerable. Voluntary contribution policies complement such UHC programs either through programs embedded in SHI—Ghana, the Kyrgyz Republic, the Philippines, and Vietnam—or through programs autonomous from SHI—India, Indonesia, Peru, Tunisia, and Turkey (before 2012). Among the countries targeting the whole informal sector, only China has a policy of voluntary contributions. The other countries in the study either exempt the nonpoor informal population from contributing (Argentina, Colombia, Mexico, and Thailand) or have developed capabilities to enforce contributory enrollment of workers in that sector and have introduced policies that make enrollment de facto mandatory for most workers in the sector—Chile, Costa Rica, and Turkey (after 2012). The mandatory approach was discussed in chapter 2, below we describe some of the experiences with voluntary contributions.

China's NRCMS was technically voluntary, targeting rural residents with generous central and local government subsidized premiums: individuals paid only 20 percent of the premium (around US$9 per person annually) with the remainder subsidized by contributions from central and local governments. Although initially the program suffered from adverse selection, population coverage rates increased following media campaigns and assessments of local authorities on their success in meeting enrollment targets (Zhang and Wang 2008).

Countries such as Ghana, Indonesia, Peru, the Philippines, and Vietnam have struggled with enrolling voluntary contributory nonpoor informal sector beneficiaries despite heavy premium subsidies. Taking some examples: in Ghana's UHC program, enrollment for those in the informal sector not already included in the exempt categories was not mandatory; the coverage rate was low and premium contributions from this population subgroup accounted for only 4 percent of UHC program revenues (see table 4.4). An estimated 80 percent of Ghana's population was in the informal sector, and only about a fifth of those were covered by the UHC program despite a steep premium subsidy: annual premiums for the informal sector were about US$10 per member, or about one-fourth the average UHC program expenditures per member of US$39 (Schieber et al. 2012).

In Peru, those in the nonpoor informal sector can join the UHC program, but less than 2 percent of all UHC program beneficiaries are from this group (Seinfeld, Montanez, and Besich 2013). In the Kyrgyz Republic, informal sector workers must pay US$10 a year to enroll, but this subgroup was not a significant source of revenues for the UHC program.

The Philippines NHIP has five different membership groups: the Employed Sector Program (for formal public and private sector workers); the Overseas Workers Program; the Individually Paying Program (IPP); the Sponsored Program (for the indigent); and the Non-Paying program (for retirees). The IPP is contributory and designed to cover those who are self-employed and in the informal sector not already covered under other programs (Manasan 2011). Enrollment in IPP is encouraged, but is not mandatory. Only about a third of the eligible population is enrolled under IPP, and members constitute about 17 percent of all NHIP enrollees and 11 percent of contributions.

Vietnam, too, has found it hard to enroll the nonpoor informal sector via voluntary contributions. Almost 75 percent of its labor force are informal, and only 60 percent have coverage (Bitran 2013). Financing for the UHC program varies by population subgroup: civil servants and formal sector workers (compulsory contributions), pensioners (social health insurer–subsidized), meritorious persons, children under six, the poor (fully government-subsidized), and the near-poor and students (partially government-subsidized). The UHC program also has a voluntary contributory component for other population groups. About 30 percent of those covered are voluntary participants, either partially subsidized (two-thirds) or from the voluntary contributory group (one-third). About 32 million people are not covered by the UHC program: almost half of them are the nonpoor working in the informal sector, about one-fourth uncovered near-poor and student groups, and the rest from populations for which full subsidies would be available. Low quality of primary care, high premiums (despite subsidies), and relatively high copayments at health facilities seem to have dissuaded people from voluntarily enrolling (Bitran 2013).

Sharing Costs—Low Copayments but Still-High OOPE

To improve access and enhance financial protection, OOPE on health has to be reduced and financing from pooled sources raised. Such spending by households not only comprises sanctioned direct payments but also captures informal payments at health facilities and beneficiaries' forced spending due to poor supply-side readiness (such as paying out of pocket for drugs at a private pharmacy because of stock-outs at public facilities).

High OOPE deters utilization (especially for the poor), risks making poor or deepening current impoverishment of households, and is a generally inequitable and regressive means of financing health systems (Ke et al. 2003; Wagstaff and van Doorslaer 2003). As countries become richer, they typically move from OOPE to pooled financing for health, undergoing a "health financing transition" (Fan and Savedoff 2014). When the OOPE share of total health expenditures is 20 percent or less, the incidence of catastrophic health expenditures and health spending-related impoverishment usually becomes negligible (WHO 2010).

Direct payments at point of service are sometimes justified from a moral hazard perspective, to limit unnecessary use of high-end services, but even then, any negative impact on equity of access to health care needs to be mitigated. About half the UHC programs reported requiring some cost sharing by beneficiaries at the point of service and, in most cases, these copayments were retained by facilities rather than pooled at a higher level.[8] The UHC programs have three types of cost sharing, each with their own rationale that are not necessarily mutually exclusive (box 4.3).

BOX 4.3
Three Cost-Sharing Modalities in UNICO Countries

The first modality appears motivated by program-protective cost containment, with caps on benefits, either budgetary amounts or quantitative restrictions designed to protect aggregate UHC program expenditures. Examples include China, India, Georgia, and Vietnam, all of which had ceilings on total amounts reimbursed from insurance programs. China's UHC program capped reimbursements at a multiple (six times) of local county or municipality income. Georgia had caps on reimbursements by service type, although these were also quite high relative to income, at around US$10,000 per operation and US$7,500 for radiation/chemotherapy. India's RSBY had an annual cap of US$500 per family beyond which families had to pay out of pocket; the RA had a higher cap: US$3,000 per family per year. Vietnam had a per episode cap of 40 months of the minimum monthly salary (about US$35 per episode per member). Other countries implemented quantitative limits: Brazil's UHC program had explicit caps on inpatient admission rates by state.

The second type seems to aim at keeping costs down by managing beneficiary utilization. Georgia's UHC program, for example, required copayments for outpatient drugs. Jamaica's program required beneficiary cost sharing at different subsidy levels for NCD drug coverage. In Kenya, outpatient curative care required a fixed copayment amount of KSH10 per contact at a dispensary and KSH20 per contact at a health center (some services, including those for pregnant women and for children under five, were exempt). In the Kyrgyz Republic, primary care was free for everyone, although most inpatient care required copayments. Beneficiaries in Vietnam were penalized by higher copayments for bypassing lower facilities without referral: 70 percent at central, 50 percent at provincial, and 30 percent at district health facilities. Tunisia and Turkey also had copayments. In some countries, copayments were specifically levied only for high-end care: in Colombia, for instance, for surgeries, hospitalization, and diagnostic imaging.

The third modality is designed to prevent any adverse financial impact of direct payments. Eleven of the 24 UNICO countries had no explicit copayments and no budgetary or quantitative restrictions (see annex 4A). Under Colombia's UHC program, copayments were required for surgery, hospitalization, and diagnostic imaging, but were capped per visit and per year, and some disease categories and vulnerable population subgroups were exempt completely, as were indigent beneficiaries in Chile, Mexico, and Tunisia.

The UNICO exercise also collected information on cost-sharing policies for broader public-sector primary care programs across the 24 countries with a focus on four "tracer" indicators: tuberculosis (TB), routine immunization, maternity services, and diabetes (see table 3.3). None of the countries resorted to copayments or user fees for TB programs, and only a few did so for child health and deliveries (often with exemptions for the poor). Yet more than half the UHC programs had cost sharing for diabetes-related care. This bifurcation points to sensitivity in countries to trying to improve their chances of meeting the millennium development goals (MDGs), but less so for noncommunicable diseases (NCDs) such as diabetes (likely due to the misperception that the latter are diseases of the affluent).

For most UHC programs informal payments did not appear to be a huge issue, but were a problem across some primary care programs. Some respondents to the Nuts & Bolts questionnaire (appendix D) reported that not enough information was available to make a substantive conclusion either way. Only one country—Ghana—noted in-kind informal payments among UHC programs. Some incidence of informal payments, often in conjunction with stock-outs, was reported for non-UHC program public-sector primary care programs in Georgia, Kenya, the Kyrgyz Republic, Mexico, Nigeria, and Peru. The relative lack of incidence of large-scale informal payments across UHC programs may represent improvements in governance, but could also be reflective of alternate mechanisms used by providers to manipulate the system (for example, in terms of inducing demand for higher-level care or gaming provider-payment mechanisms to seek higher reimbursements). Analysis of household survey data indicates that OOPE remains relatively high in some countries, even those with coverage and not requiring cost sharing (at least on paper). Deeper exploration of the reasons behind persistence in OOPE despite rising coverage—such as who is continuing with OOPE and why—is needed.

National Health Accounts data indicate that the median OOPE share of total health expenditures was about 37 percent across UNICO countries in 2011—slightly lower than the median across non-UNICO developing countries of 38 percent in the same year—and a decline of 2 percentage points from 2000. The OOPE share of total health spending remains relatively high in most UNICO countries, higher than what might be expected relative to income and relative to WHO's benchmark of 20 percent (figure 4.7). The OOPE share was highest (above 60 percent) in Georgia, Nigeria, and India. OOPE shares were below 20 percent in only four countries: South Africa, Thailand, Colombia, and Turkey.

Over 2000–12, Thailand had the fastest decline in the OOPE share of total health spending, at more than 6 percent a year. China, Turkey, South Africa, Argentina, and the Kyrgyz Republic also had relatively rapid declines, at more than 2 percent a year. Yet in nine countries the OOPE share went up over the period, notably Colombia, the Philippines, and Costa Rica (although the increase was from a low base in Colombia and Costa Rica) (figure 4.8).

With progress toward UHC, one would expect the share of OOPE to decline, and it remains a key concern why it is not occurring in more UNICO countries. Trends in OOPE represent not just the extent of financial protection accorded by UHC programs but also reflect the extent,

FIGURE 4.7

OOPE Share of Total Health Expenditures versus GDP per Capita in UNICO Countries, 2011 (UNICO countries highlighted)

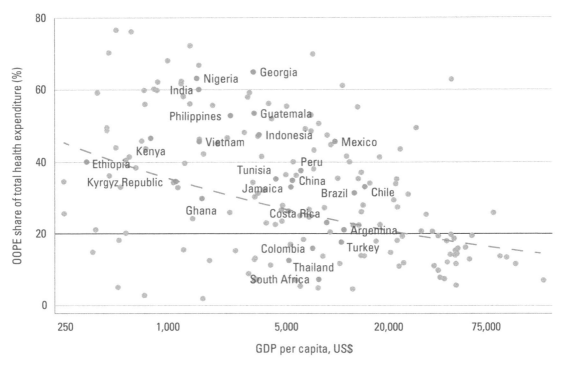

Source: World Development Indicators database.
Note: X-axis logged.

breadth, depth, and height of other coverage programs in some countries. The extent to which OOPE is catastrophic and impoverishing matters more than the level of OOPE per se: if most OOPE is made by the relatively well off, who are, perhaps, willing to pay out of pocket for better responsiveness of care, this may be less of a concern to policy makers than when high levels of OOPE reflect low or shallow coverage among the poor.

Pooling Risk and Allocating Resources

More than half of total health spending in two-thirds of UNICO countries comes from pooled sources of financing (defined in box 4.4), according to National Health Accounts data. Pooling as a share of total health spending was in 2011 lowest in Georgia, India, and Nigeria, and highest in South Africa, Colombia, Turkey, Costa Rica, and Thailand. The pooled share of total health expenditures generally climbed with income.

UNICO countries have adopted three main types of categories of risk pooling. Most SHI+/SHI++ programs are in single, national risk pools.

FIGURE 4.8

Annual Change in OOPE Share of Total Health Expenditures in UNICO Countries, 2000–12 (UNICO countries highlighted)

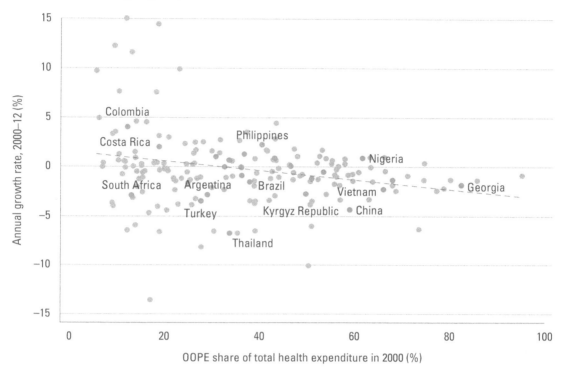

Source: World Development Indicators database.

Others, including several SSPs, PVPs, and ISPs, are separate national risk pools coexisting with one or more parallel risk pools, each covering different subgroups. Some UHC programs are embedded in multiple, subnational risk pools.

Single, National Risk Pools

Programs in the first group include four of the six SHI+/SHI++ programs and one PVP: Costa Rica, Ghana, Georgia, the Kyrgyz Republic, and the Philippines.[9] As a share of national population covered, Costa Rica had the largest single-payer program among UNICO countries. Its noncontributory UHC program component (providing coverage for about 12 percent of the national population) is part of a single, national pool that covers about 91 percent of the population) (Escobar, Griffin, and Shaw 2010). The single pools of the Philippines and the Kyrgyz Republic cover large shares of the population (83 percent and 76 percent). Ghana's UHC program combines resources into a single national pool, although population coverage

---

BOX 4.4
Pooling Risk

Risk pooling is the mechanism by which revenues are aggregated in order to spread financial risk associated with health expenditures across individuals and over time. Pooling is the "insurance" function of financing: pooled revenues are used to pay for health care needs of individuals, reducing or eliminating the need for OOPE at the point and time of service.

Pooling enables the replacement of large, unpredictable OOPE on health with a stream of smaller, predictable prepayments (paid through general taxation or insurance premiums). Depending on how the contributions and allocations are structured, pooling can allow for improvements in the efficiency and equity of health financing by providing a mechanism for resources to be allocated according to an individual's health care needs, reducing the uncertainty that he or she faces on health-related expenditure, and redistributing resources to the poor (Smith and Witter 2004).

Key pooling considerations are size, composition, and number of risk pools, and the extent to which pooling allows for cross-subsidization. Larger, more diverse risk pools generally have the advantage of greater predictability and lower variations in expected health spending, reducing financial uncertainty for individuals and providers (WHO 2000). Fragmented pools, in contrast, tend to have higher administrative costs and shallower benefit coverage. Unified risk pools may also help to control expenditures due to monopsony power and to minimize adverse selection (Results for Development Institute 2011).

(33 percent) is much lower than that of most of the other single-pool countries. Georgia's MIP—covering about 20 percent of the population—is also technically a single national pool, albeit one that does not have any contributory members as it is financed purely by the central government.[10]

Separate National Risk Pools with One or More Parallel Risk Pools

Programs in the second group include Chile's UHC program (Fonasa), an SHI++, alongside seven for-profit private insurers (known as *Isapres*) with the latter covering about one-sixth of the population. Kenya's UHC program—the Health Sector Services Fund—allocates government- and donor-financed resources directly to health facilities, and a parallel, mandatory risk pool for formal sector workers—the National Hospital Insurance Fund—finances health care in public and private facilities for 18 percent of Kenyans. Peru's UHC program (SIS) and Tunisia's UHC program (Free Medical Assistance for the Poor) exist as parallel risk pools additional to national SHI programs: EsSalud in Peru and Caisse Nationale de l'Assurance Maladie (CNAM) in Tunisia. Thailand's UHC program (UCS) covers 71 percent of the population using central government revenues; it coexists with two additional prominent risk pools: the Compulsory Social Security Scheme that covers private formal employees and the Civil Servant Medical Benefit Scheme that covers public formal employees (table 4.6).

Multiple, Subnational Risk Pools

The third category has subnational risk pools, typically augmented by financing from the central government, with or without additional parallel risk pools (table 4.7). For example, Argentina's UHC program, Plan

TABLE 4.6
National Pools and Selected Parallel Risk Pools, 2011

Country	Risk-pooling program	Primary target population	Share of national population covered (%)
Chile	UHC program: Fonasa	Poor; formal, informal sector	78
	Isapres	High income	17
Guatemala	UHC program: Expansion of Coverage Program	Poor areas	29
	MoH	National	71
	Guatemala Social Security Institute	Formal sector	18
Jamaica	UHC program: National Health Fund	NCD patients; elderly	19
	MoH	National	100
Kenya	UHC program: Health Sector Services Fund	National	48
	National Hospital Insurance Fund	Formal, informal sector	18
Peru	UHC program: Seguro Integral de Salud	Poor	43
	EsSalud	Formal sector	29
Thailand	UHC program: Universal Coverage Scheme	Uninsured	71
	Compulsory Social Security Scheme	Formal private sector	13
	Civil Servant Medical Benefit Scheme	Formal public sector	8
Tunisia	UHC program: Free Medical Assistance for the Poor	Poor; near-poor	27
	Caisse Nationale de l'Assurance Maladie	Formal sector	68

Source: UNICO studies.
Note: UNICO UHC programs in bold. Totals may not add up to 100% because of lack of full coverage, other smaller insurance programs, and overlapping coverage.

TABLE 4.7
Multiple Subnational Risk Pools and Selected Parallel Risk-Pooling Programs

Country	UHC program	Subnational UHC program risk pool	Primary target population	Share of national population covered (%)
Argentina	UHC program: Plan Nacer	Province	Uninsured pregnant; children <6	4
	National Social Health Insurance Organizations		Formal sector	47
	Institute of Social Services for Retirees and Pensioners		Pensioners	8
	Provincial Health Insurance Organizations		Provincial public sector	14
Brazil	UHC program: Family Health Strategy	Municipality	National	100
	Sistema Suplementar de Saúde		Formal sector; high income	25
China	UHC program: New Rural Cooperative Medical Scheme	County	Rural	62
	Urban Resident Basic Medical Insurance		Informal sector; students; urban	19
Colombia	UHC program: Subsidized Regime	Municipality	Poor; near poor; informal sector	52
	Contributory Regime		Formal sector; high income	47
India	UHC program: National Rural Health Mission	State	Rural	70
	UHC program: Rashtriya Swasthya Bima Yojna	State	Poor	6
	UHC program: Rajiv Aarogyasri	State	Poor; near poor	6
Mexico	UHC program: Seguro Popular	State	Uninsured	43
	Instituto Mexicano del Seguro Social		Private formal sector	35
	Instituto de Seguridad		Public formal sector	5
Vietnam	UHC program: Social Health Insurance	Provincial	National	64

Source: UNICO studies.
Note: UNICO UHC programs in bold. Totals may not add up to 100% because of lack of full coverage, other smaller insurance programs, and overlapping coverage.

Nacer, is a noncontributory ISP that blends World Bank financing via the central government with capitated transfers to 23 provinces, with pooling at provincial level, along with 24 percent of resources provided by provinces themselves to cover poor and vulnerable populations. (The program covers about 4 percent of the national population and targets poor, uninsured households with pregnant women, children under six years of age, women who have recently delivered or miscarried, and indigenous populations.) Plan Nacer operates in a fragmented health financing system with several additional parallel risk pools: the National Social Health Insurance Organizations covering formal workers and their dependents (47 percent of the population); the Institute of Social Services for Retirees and Pensioners (8 percent); and Provincial Health Insurance Organizations covering provincial public employees (14 percent).

Pooling for Brazil's UHC program is among the more than 5,000 municipalities, and so a complex, fragmented parallel system of private insurers covers the formal public and private sectors, providing coverage for about 25 percent of the national population.

Colombia's Subsidized Regime also pools at municipal level and coexists with a parallel risk pool, the Contributory Regime. Pooling in India's and Mexico's UHC programs is at state level. China's NRCMS is pooled at county level.[11] Vietnam's UHC program operates with provincial risk pools.

Cross-Subsidizing the Poor? Yes and No

The advantages of SHI+/SHI++ programs on cross-subsidization were evident (and assessed) in some countries, less clear in others. For example, Costa Rica's pooled expenditures were progressive: the poorest 20 percent of the population received at least 30 percent of pooled expenditure benefits, the wealthiest 20 percent only some 11 percent. In Ghana the incidence of VAT was mildly progressive (Akazili et al. 2012). The country's UHC program contributions by the formal sector were also progressive, but voluntary prepayments by those in the informal sector were regressive: the incidence of benefits of health care services was generally pro-rich, except for utilization of inpatient services at district hospitals. The distribution of benefits across primary care was relatively evenly shared across economic quintiles (Akazili et al. 2012).

Under Jamaica's UHC program, even though the program has increased overall utilization and reduced NCD-related OOPE, the rich have benefited more from government subsidies than the poor, and inequality in access has increased. Part of the reason is the lack of targeting of the poor in the UHC program: eligibility is determined by age and NCD incidence, not by economic status.

The fragmentation or otherwise of the risk pools seems to have little bearing on equity gains. Although theoretically the benefits of single risk pools should outweigh those of fragmented systems, several UNICO countries that have expanded coverage and improved health system outcomes in the past decade have done so without single, national pools (including Colombia, Mexico, and Thailand). Some countries with single risk pools, however, have adjusted benefits to favor contributory members, limiting equity gains from cross-subsidization and harmonization.[12]

Other countries have explicitly cross-subsidized despite fragmented risk pools, including Colombia, Jamaica, and Tunisia. All three earmark contributions of parallel risk pools to finance coverage for the poor. In Colombia, Contributory Regime members finance 41 percent of the resources for the Subsidized Regime. A similar earmark helps finance Jamaica's UHC program, providing a cross-subsidy in terms of health but not economic status. Tunisia's UHC program, as well as full government subsidization, has indirect cross-subsidization from the parallel formal risk pool (CNAM, worth 20 percent of UHC program revenues) and from OOPE by near-poor enrollees (10 percent); the rest is covered by the central government.

Fiscal Transfers and Resource Allocations across Levels of Care

Allocations of pooled resources down subnational administrative units and across levels of care can be designed to enhance equity. They can also enhance the technical and allocative efficiency of pooled funds (by, for example, delineating an optimal mix going to preventive or promotive versus curative or rehabilitative care). Yet such allocations may introduce or exacerbate current rigidities (such as inequitable geographic distribution of health facilities) that block resources from flowing to where they are needed most. For health-specific transfers, countries often use a combination of several proxy measures to allocate resources based on relative need, including population size; demographics (young children, the elderly, and women of child-bearing age tend to need and use health care more than other subgroups); levels of ill-health (with mortality rates used as proxies); and socioeconomic status (poorer subgroups tend to need more health care and are more reliant on public financing) (McIntyre 2007).

Most UNICO countries have decentralized health systems (table 4.8), yet the source of financing for most UHC programs is central government (see table 4.4). Even among countries that are fiscally decentralized, subnational own-source revenues are almost always lower than subnational expenditures, necessitating central government financing to bridge the

TABLE 4.8

Centralized versus Decentralized Health Care Provision in UNICO Countries

Central level	First-tier level	Second- or lower-tier level
Costa Rica; Georgia; Kenya[a]	Argentina; India; Jamaica; Mexico; Peru; South Africa; Tunisia; Turkey	Brazil; Chile; China; Colombia; Ethiopia; Ghana; Guatemala; Indonesia; Kyrgyz Republic; Nigeria; Philippines; Thailand; Vietnam

Source: UNICO case studies.
a. Kenya is decentralizing to county level.

gap (Boadway and Shah 2007). Hence the intergovernmental fiscal transfer mechanism by which resources are allocated to lower levels is potentially an important policy instrument. Fiscal transfers can be general or
specific purpose, the latter providing incentives for subnational governments to undertake certain activities (Boadway and Shah 2007).

UNICO countries showed no clear patterns among resource allocation
modalities. Several UHC programs transferred resources (or some por-
tion) based on simple formulas. In Colombia, for example, fiscal transfers
from the national government were made to municipalities on a capitation basis (number of poor people enrolled in the program within each
municipality. There was no adjustment for risk or for other community
characteristics. These capitated amounts were used by beneficiaries to
purchase insurance from municipal health insurance plans. Part of
financing for Indonesia's Jamkesmas was transferred to districts also on a
simple, capitated basis.

Other UHC programs transferred resources using some form of risk- or
equity-based adjustment (or both). Financing for primary care under
Chile's UHC program was based on capitated transfers to municipalities
via regional health authorities. About 60 percent of these capitated transfers were adjusted for the catchment area's age structure, sex, socioeconomic status, and rural/urban split (Ellis and Fernandez 2013). Kenya's
UHC program designed allocations to be higher for high-poverty areas
with low population density, and relatively high costs of providing services (this last adjustment yet to be made operational).

Argentina's Plan Nacer provides capitated payments (about US$48 a
year per beneficiary enrolled) to provinces, which are then used to purchase services from providers. Given that the program targets the poor
and uninsured, allocations to provinces with a greater number of these
targeted subgroups are probably higher. There is also an added incentive for provinces to enroll targeted individuals because 70 percent of the
capitated amount is financed by donors via the national government.
In addition, Plan Nacer transfers resources to provinces based partly on

results: 60 percent of the total capitated amount is paid when beneficiaries enroll; a further 40 percent only after verification that provinces have reached targets for 10 tracer MCH indicators at provincial level. This mechanism also aims to enhance accountability (a theme picked up in chapter 6).

Transfers from the federal government to municipalities for cofinancing Brazil's UHC program, as in Argentina, are also made in two parts: a fixed per capita amount and a variable part linked to attaining targets for coverage and services (for example, the number of Family Health Service teams active in each municipality or state).

Guatemala makes annual capitation payments to jurisdictions (each of roughly 10,000 people) of around US$6–9: it gives higher amounts to jurisdictions in priority municipalities and those with higher chronic malnutrition rates among the target population; it makes disbursements quarterly, based on performance measured by 28 indicators of service provision (such as immunization coverage and utilization of maternal health care services).

Yet fiscal transfers in some countries have sustained, not mitigated, inequities. Vietnam is one example. Each of its 63 provinces receives UHC program funds that are capped at 90 percent of the membership-related contributions in that province, which means that, Hanoi and Ho Chi Minh City apart, provincial expenditures are always less than provincial revenues for the remaining 61 provinces. Below provincial level, funds are transferred based on a complex combination of group-specific capitation and historical utilization rates, all of which create barriers to reallocating funds to where needs are greatest.

Many UNICO countries differentiated payment mechanisms for primary versus hospital-based care, but it was unclear whether resources were earmarked across levels of care. In the Kyrgyz Republic, primary care payments were capitation-based whereas hospital-based payments were case-based by clinical cost group, a form of the DRG payment modality. Although not ring-fenced at the outset, primary care accounted for 40 percent of total UHC program expenditures in that country.

In some UHC programs earmarking was clearly stated in terms of shares of resources for different levels of care. In China's NRCMS, for example, a fixed share of total resources (20–30 percent depending on municipality) was dedicated to outpatient care. A small share of China's NRCMS direct contributions was also ring-fenced for use by households to cover outpatient services. In Indonesia, the Jamkesmas premium was separated for use by primary or by secondary and tertiary care: 15 percent was set aside for primary care and transferred to district health offices, with retrospective utilization-based accounting; the balance covered hospital-based care with reimbursements being made using a form of DRG.

Conclusions and Policy Implications

UHC program expenditures per beneficiary in 2011 were strongly corre-lated with GDP per capita, with lower-income UNICO countries generally spending less per beneficiary. Such expenditures were higher for UHC programs embedded in SHI programs. Most UHC program expenditures do not appear excessive because they operate as discrete demand-side additions to publicly financed supply-side financing and, in some cases, are complemented by private OOPE (by design).

In other words, most UHC program expenditures are incremental and on their own do not reflect the full cost of coverage. Therefore, in assess-ing the fiscal sustainability of UHC programs, one key implication is the importance of taking a more holistic systems view of health financing rather than a narrow program view. In this light, the fiscal outlays associ-ated with UHC expansions are higher than what an assessment of pro-gram expenditures alone would suggest, but still not excessive relative to income comparators: in 2011, the median UHC program spending per beneficiary across UNICO countries was US$39, about 1.4 percent of GDP per capita and 0.4 percent of GDP.

The above analysis confirms the importance of government financ-ing in expanding coverage for the poor: some 70 percent of revenues across all UHC programs come from general government revenues. Coverage for the poor, whether targeted or part of a universal program, was noncontributory in all UNICO UHC programs. Half the UNICO countries had diverse forms of earmarked taxes to cofinance coverage expansions.

With few exceptions, voluntary contributions from the nonpoor informal sector are not a prominent source of finance for coverage expan-sion. By contrast, OOPE by households still is, sometimes deliberately so on the grounds that copayments limit "unnecessary" utilization. Beyond that the OOPE share in total health expenditure is high in many UNICO countries, suggesting that a greater focus on improving the height of cov-erage in the UHC cube is needed.

A focus on equity is already apparent in risk pooling. As most UHC programs are not part of national, single-payer pools, many governments have made risk- and equity-based adjustments in intergovernmental fis-cal allocations. Others have used matching and results-based allocations to enhance the resource base and effectiveness of UHC program financ-ing. Some evidence of ring-fencing of allocations across levels of care is also evident, although more information is needed.

Some good health-financing practices stand out. UHC programs that provide comprehensive coverage and are embedded within single-program UHC initiatives provide several potential advantages for reducing fragmentation, promoting solidarity, and enabling cross-subsidization. Still, several countries have expanded coverage without following a single risk-pool model, including Colombia, Mexico, and Thailand. Others, such as Chile via its AUGE reform, have attempted to harmonize benefits without necessarily pooling financing, or, like Colombia, Jamaica, and Tunisia, have explicitly cross-subsidized financing across risk pools without merging them.

When expanding coverage, some countries such as Argentina and Thailand have covered the informal sector using fully subsidized government financing, overcoming a major revenue-collection challenge in attaining UHC and moving to the equity-enhancing objective. A very few countries, notably China, appear to have had a measure of success in enrolling informal nonpoor populations that are making voluntary contributions, but whether this is easily replicable in other political systems is open to question. The relative lack of dependence on external financing for expanding coverage is also notable as it potentially signals strong domestic political commitments. Good practices are evident in some countries that tie intergovernmental resource allocations to attainment of results (as in Argentina).

The analysis of financing information gleaned from the UNICO countries underscores several key policy implications.

Appreciating the Overall Macro-Fiscal Context and Financial Sustainability

Given reliance on government sources for financing poor-focused expansions, there has to be a greater understanding of the macro-fiscal context of health financing, including potential sources of additional government spending for health, and its prioritization. The move toward making benefit packages more explicit potentially exposes countries to fiscal sustainability risks—for example, from cost pressures, increased utilization rates, and adoption of expensive medicines and technology in the future—especially as accountability mechanisms mature in countries that lag behind. Some UNICO countries have mitigated fiscal sustainability risks by explicitly limiting or circumscribing benefits. For example, in 2011 programs in Argentina and Nigeria covered only MCH benefits. Chile's AUGE program is another example where a new policy legally required that all social insurance programs deliver preventive and curative health guarantees for a minimum set of priority diseases based on clear treatment protocols, within specific time limits, and with copayment ceilings;

further, the guarantee is for a subset of procedures that have an estimated cost that is less than the total budget, giving the UHC program
some cushion.

Looming Fiscal Sustainability Risks in Some Countries

These are the countries that have promised open-ended comprehensive
entitlements that are not explicit and are, in effect, not universally made
available to all beneficiaries, thus leading to implicit rationing that disproportionately affects the poor and vulnerable. Short term, the fiscal risks
in such countries may be low if this implicit rationing continues, but
longer term, benefits may need to be made more explicit to mitigate sustainability challenges.

Ensuring Complementary Demand- and Supply-Side Financing

Although most UHC programs provide demand-side financing, many also
feature traditional supply-side financing and cofinancing of public health
facilities. This strongly suggests that policy stipulations are needed for
flexibility and leveraging in using demand-side funds to attain UHC
objectives, combined with strong accountability mechanisms (chapter 6).

Enrolling the Nonpoor Informal Sector

Some UNICO countries appear to have enrolled many of the nonpoor
informal sector via a contributory modality. More information is needed
as to how this was managed and implemented, and whether any specific
strategies used can yield lessons.

Understanding the Persistence of OOPE

More research is needed on the extent to which OOPE reflects inadequate financing for UHC and poor supply-side readiness, and on height-
of-coverage issues.

Sensitizing Policy to Progressivity and Cross-Subsidization

The diversity of pooling and resource allocation across UNICO countries
underscores the need for policy to be sensitive to issues of progressivity of
financing sources and awareness of the extent of cross-subsidization in
pooled funds across UHC programs.

Annex 4A

Country	Name of UHC program	UHC program spending share of GDP (%)	Coverage (millions)	Share of national population (%)	Benefit package	Cost sharing	UHC program spending share of public health expenditure (%)
Nigeria	National Health Insurance Scheme	0.001	1.2	0.8	MCH	No	0.04
Argentina	Plan Nacer	0.02	1.7	4	MCH	No	0.3
Kenya	Health Sector Services Fund	0.02	20	48	Primary	Yes	0.9
Guatemala	Expansion of Coverage Program	0.1	4.4	29	Primary	No	2.6
Indonesia	Jamkesmas	0.1	76.4	32	Comprehensive	No	7.0
Peru	Seguro Integral de Salud	0.1	12.7	42	Comprehensive	No	4.3
India	National Rural Health Mission	0.16	840	70	Primary	No	13.5
India	Rashtriya Swasthya Bima Yojna	0.01	70	6	Secondary	Yes, caps	0.5
India	Rajiv Aarogyasri	0.01	70	6	Tertiary	Yes, caps	1.0
South Africa	Antiretroviral Treatment Program	0.2	1.5	3	HIV/AIDS	No	5.0
Turkey	Green Card	0.3	9.1	12	Comprehensive	Yes	5.8
Jamaica	Jamaica National Health Fund	0.4	0.5	19	NCD drugs	Yes	13.4

table continues next page

ANNEX 4A *(Continued)*

Country	Name of UHC program	UHC program spending share of GDP (%)	Coverage (millions)	Share of national population (%)	Benefit package	Cost sharing	UHC program spending share of public health expenditure (%)
Philippines	National Health Insurance Fund	0.4	78.4	83	Comprehensive	Yes	26.5
Tunisia	Free Medical Assistance for the Poor	0.4	3	27	Comprehensive	Yes, for nonpoor enrollees	13.7
Mexico	Seguro Popular	0.5	51.8	43	Comprehensive	Yes, for nonpoor enrollees	18.0
Georgia	Medical Insurance Program	0.6	0.9	20	Comprehensive	Yes	36.5
China	New Rural Cooperative Medical Scheme	0.8	832	64	Comprehensive	Yes	22.2
Ethiopia	Health Extension Program	0.8	60.9	68	Primary	No	4.3
Vietnam	Social Health Insurance	0.9	55.4	63	Comprehensive	Yes	35.9
Ghana	National Health Insurance Scheme	1.0	8.2	33	Comprehensive	No	33.0
Brazil	Family Health Strategy	1.1	200	100	Primary	Yes, caps	26.2
Colombia	Subsidized Regime	1.2	22.3	47	Comprehensive	Yes, for nonpoor enrollees	24.0
Thailand	Universal Coverage Scheme	1.2	47.7	71	Comprehensive	No	40.1

table continues next page

ANNEX 4A *(Continued)*

Country	Name of UHC program	UHC program spending share of GDP (%)	Coverage (millions)	Share of national population (%)	Benefit package	Cost sharing	UHC program spending share of public health expenditure (%)
Kyrgyz Republic	Mandatory Health Insurance Fund	1.8	4.2	76	Comprehensive	Yes	48.5
Chile	Fonasa	2.1	13.2	78	Comprehensive	Yes, for nonpoor enrollees	56.5
Costa Rica	Caja Costarricense de Seguridad Social	6.2	4.3	91	Comprehensive	No	81.0
Median		*0.4*	*16.6*	*42.5*			*13.6*

Source: UNICO studies.

Notes

1. Provider payment mechanisms—a component of purchasing under the financing function of health systems—are discussed in chapter 3.
2. It is not always clear how much a country should spend on health and what constitutes "low" or "high" expenditures (see Savedoff 2007). Nevertheless, benchmarking can be one guide: for example, high-income Organisation for Economic Co-operation and Development (OECD) countries, almost all of which are closer to attaining UHC than UNICO countries, spend an average of 10 percent of GDP on health; others recommend a benchmark of at least 5 percent of GDP.
3. Table A2.7 gives coverage rates for programs.
4. The median health share of the government budget in high-income countries was 12.9 percent in 2011.
5. As discussed in chapter 6, some countries have been more active leveraging this potential (including Argentina, Brazil, and Guatemala) than others.
6. The subnational government financing share was highest in Brazil's UHC program, in which 64 percent of revenues came from municipal governments and a further 10 percent from state governments.
7. The Philippines has also recently introduced earmarked taxes on alcohol and tobacco to finance its UHC program; Vietnam is also considering introducing an earmarked tobacco tax for financing part of its UHC program.
8. See annex 4A for cost-sharing modalities across UHC programs.

9. Turkey (2012) and Indonesia (2014) have since instituted single-payer UHC programs by merging social insurance schemes.
10. Georgia has since expanded coverage to its entire population.
11. China has five levels of government administration: central, provincial, prefecture, county, and town. It has 330 prefectures and 2,600 counties.
12. In Indonesia, for example, although medical benefits are the same for all, contributory members have access to better hospital rooms and can choose empaneled private providers for primary care.

References

ADB (Asian Development Bank). 2012. *Tobacco Taxes: A Win-Win Measure for Fiscal Space and Health*. Manila: ADB.

Akazili, J., B. Garshong, M. Aikins, J. Gyapong, and D. McIntyre. 2012. "Progressivity of Health Care Financing and Incidence of Service Benefits in Ghana." *Health Policy and Planning* 27: 113–22.

Bitran, R. 2013. "Universal Health Coverage and the Challenge of Informal Employment: Lessons from Developing Countries." HNP Discussion Paper, World Bank, Washington, DC.

Boadway, R., and A. Shah, eds. 2007. *Intergovernmental Fiscal Transfers: Principles and Practice*. Washington, DC: World Bank.

Buchanan, J. M. 1963. "The Economics of Earmarked Taxes." *Journal of Political Economy* 71 (5): 457–69.

Cabrera, E. C. T. 2011. "Colombia: The Subsidized Health-Care Scheme in the Social Protection System." In *Successful Social Protection Floor Experiences*. Vol 18 of series Sharing Innovative Experiences. New York: United Nations Development Programme.

Cichon, M., W. Newbrander, H. Yamabana, A. Weber, et al. 1999. *Modelling in Health Care Finance: A Compendium of Quantitative Techniques for Health Care Financing*. Geneva: International Labour Office.

Ellis, R. P., and J. G. Fernandez. 2013. "Risk Selection, Risk Adjustment and Choice: Concepts and Lessons from the Americas." *International Journal of Environmental Research and Public Health* 10: 5299–332.

Escobar, M., C. Griffin, and R. P. Shaw. 2010. *The Impact of Health Insurance in Low- and Middle-Income Countries*. Washington, DC: Brookings Institution Press.

Fan, V. Y., and W. D. Savedoff. 2014. "The Health Financing Transition: A Conceptual Framework and Empirical Evidence." *Social Science and Medicine* 105: 115–21.

Gottret, P., and G. Schieber. 2006. *Health Financing Revisited: A Practitioner's Guide*. Washington, DC: World Bank.

Grover, A. 2011. "Report of the Special Rapporteur on the Right of Everyone to the Enjoyment of the Highest Attainable Standard of Physical and Mental Health." United Nations Human Rights Council, Geneva.

Hsiao, W. C. 2007. "Why Is a Systematic View of Health Financing Necessary?" *Health Affairs* 26 (4): 950–61.

Ke, Xu, D. B. Evans, K. Kawabata, R Zeramdini, et al. 2003. "Household Catastrophic Health Expenditure: A Multicountry Analysis." *The Lancet* 362 (9378): 111–17.

Kutzin, J., C. Cashin, and M. Jakab, eds. 2010. *Implementing Health Financing Reforms: Lessons from Countries in Transition*. Brussels: European Observatory on Health Systems and Policies.

Manasan, R. G. 2011. "Expanding Social Health Insurance Coverage: New Issues and Challenges." Discussion Paper Series 2011–21, Philippine Institute for Development Studies, Makati City.

McIntyre, D. 2007. *Learning from Experience: Health Care Financing in Low- and Middle-Income Countries*. Geneva: Global Forum for Health Research.

McLeary, W. 1991. "The Earmarking of Government Revenue: A Review of Some World Bank Experience." *The World Bank Research Observer* 6 (1): 81–104.

Murray, C. J. L. M., and A. Tandon. 2008. "Purchasing Power Parity Comparison in Health." *ICP Bulletin* 5 (1): 41–43.

Prakongsai, P., W. Patcharanarumol, and V. Tangcharoensathien. 2008. "Can Earmarking Mobilize and Sustain Resources to the Health Sector?" *Bulletin of the World Health Organization* 86 (11): 898–901.

Results for Development Institute. 2011. *Should India Create a Single National Risk Pool? Some Lessons from Thailand, Mexico, and Colombia*. Washington, DC: Results for Development Institute.

Savedoff, W. D. 2007. "What Should a Country Spend on Health Care?" *Health Affairs* 26 (4): 962–70.

Schiavo-Campo, S. 2007. "The Budget and Its Coverage." In *Budgeting and Budgetary Institutions*, edited by A. Shah, 53–88. Washington, DC: World Bank.

Schieber, G., C. Cashin, K. Saleh, and R. Lavado. 2012. *Health Financing in Ghana*. Washington, DC: World Bank.

Seinfeld, J., V. Montanez, and N. Besich. 2013. *The Health Insurance System in Peru: Towards a Universal Health Insurance*. New Delhi: Global Development Network.

Smith, P. C., and S. N. Witter. 2004. "Risk Pooling in Health Care Financing: Implications for Health System Performance." HNP Discussion Paper, World Bank, Washington, DC.

Van Tien, T., H. T. Phuong, I. Mathauer, and N. T. K. Phuong. 2011. *A Health Financing Review of Viet Nam with a Focus on Social Health Insurance*. Hanoi: World Health Organization.

Wagstaff, A., and E. van Doorslaer. 2003. "Catastrophe and Impoverishment in Paying for Health Care: With Applications to Vietnam 1993–1998." *Health Economics* 12: 921–34.

Wagstaff, A. 2010. "Social Health Insurance Reexamined." *Health Economics* 19: 503–17.

Wang, H., K. Switlick, C. Ortiz, B. Zurita, and C. Connor. 2012. *Health Insurance Handbook: How to Make It Work?* Washington, DC: World Bank.

WHO (World Health Organization). 2000. *World Health Report 2000: Health Systems—Improving Performance.* Geneva: WHO.

———. 2010. *Monitoring the Building Blocks of Health Systems: A Handbook of Indicators and Their Measurement Strategies.* Geneva: WHO.

Zhang, L., and H. Wang. 2008. "Dynamic Process of Adverse Selection: Evidence from Subsidized Community-Based Health Insurance in Rural China." *Social Science and Medicine* 67 (7): 1173–82.

CHAPTER 5

Improving Health Care Provision

Introduction

Better-managed money and more financial resources may indeed be required for universal health coverage (UHC), but alone they are not enough to deliver high-quality health care services. The health care provision system has to be able to deliver the services for affordable access to the needed health care services in the right spot as coverage expands. Even if a country has a well-defined and financed health coverage program with well-identified beneficiaries, it cannot achieve its intended results without a well-organized health care provision system that can respond to the demand.

In this chapter we describe five areas of intervention commonly pursued alongside the UHC programs in Universal Health Coverage Studies Series (UNICO) countries to expand health care services provision, from which we draw a few policy implications.

Human Resources for Health—Trends in Retention and Outreach

UHC programs are designed to close a financing gap and a provision gap. Some of the provision gap facing the poor and vulnerable populations in UNICO countries results from the distance, physical and cultural, between health workers and the populations they serve—a gap that countries are aiming to bridge with retention incentives for rural areas and with community health workers (CHWs).

The current density of health workers in urban and rural areas varies widely across UNICO countries (figure 5.1). Countries in Africa had the lowest density with an average of 1.03 health workers per 1,000 people, against 2.82 among the 24 UNICO countries as a whole. Countries and regions also show wide variations internally of course, especially between urban and rural areas. Although most countries have increased their human resources over the past couple of decades, density has stagnated in some countries such as Ethiopia, Nigeria, and South Africa, and even fallen in others, including Ghana, India, Jamaica, and Peru. World Health Organization (WHO) recommends 2.28 health workers per 1,000 people, though some studies suggest that a still higher ratio may be needed to expand population-based health care services. Regression results from 18 Sub-Saharan African countries suggest that this number of health workers would only achieve 50 percent coverage for Pap smear tests, 20 percent for HIV tests during pregnancy and pelvic exams, and less than 10 percent for mammograms (Soucat, Scheffler, and Ghebreyesus 2013). Analysis of low- and middle-income countries also reveals that, although the density of doctors and nurses was positively associated with skilled birth attendance and measles immunization rates,

FIGURE 5.1
Density of Health Workers in UNICO Countries

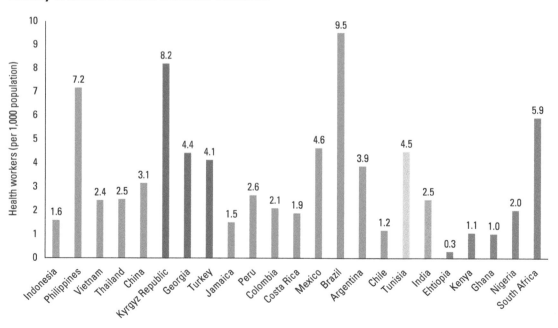

Source: WHO Global Health Observatory. Data represent the latest data available after 2004.
Note: Health workers refer to the sum of physicians, nursing, and midwifery personnel. Countries are sorted first by region, then income level measured by GDP per capita.

it did not account for variations in postnatal care coverage, TB detection, Cesarean section, or clinic visits of children with acute respiratory infections (Kruk et al. 2010), indicating more to human resources than this aggregate number alone.

Distribution issues, too, need to be resolved, especially that health workers are available in rural and remote areas. Most UHC programs use a combination of policies to create incentives for health care providers to work in rural areas and with vulnerable populations. Twenty-two of the 24 UNICO countries have programs that encourage or requires doctors and other health workers to spend part of their career in poor and or rural areas. In 13 of the countries the program involves financial incentives, which in some countries can be high; in Indonesia the premium can be 250% of the base salary. In India the NRHM allows fee-for-service payments (for anesthetists, for instance) to contract private medical professionals to serve public facilities in rural areas. In 12 countries there are increased career opportunities linked to serving in these areas. In seven countries rural service is a precondition for a public sector job. Also to attract doctors to rural areas, some UHC programs improve the attraction of rural location for health workers by offering nonmonetary incentives, such as better work conditions, and training and conference support. In Nigeria, for example, where no direct payment is made for health care providers' performance, added revenues for the health facilities arising out of the UHC program have made it possible to improve the working environment, helping lift health workers' welfare and productivity. Finally, in seven countries, service in rural locations is a requisite for graduating from medical school.

UNICO countries have adopted outreach services involving trained and supervised CHWs—usually recruited from the same communities they serve in. CHWs are in use both in dispersed populations (as in Ethiopia and Guatemala) and in dense urban settings (as in Brazil, India, Nigeria, and Peru). They are deployed to improve the link between primary-health-care (PHC) and catchment populations by voicing their collective needs and facilitating access to prevention, care, and follow-up treatment. These workers help providers better respond to changing socioeconomic, demographic, and epidemiological needs. They are also designed to move away from a system of "conventional care" marked by a relationship limited to the moment of consultation and with a focus on illness, to a "people-centered" model. This model is marked by an enduring personal relationship with a focus on health care needs, reflecting a mission of responsibility for health of all in the community along the life cycle, tackling determinants of ill health, and maintaining health.

In Brazil, each FHS team consists of one general practitioner, one nurse, two nursing assistants, up to 12 community agents (each community agent is responsible for a maximum of 750 individuals) and, in some cases, dental health professionals. The community agents have played a key role in the successful outreach efforts of this program. In Costa Rica, a team formed by a physician, a nurse, and a primary care technical assistant provides promotive, preventive, and curative services while serving as a link in the referral chain to other levels of care. In Guatemala, the PEC, particularly in rural and remote areas, contracted nongovernmental organizations to provide services using mobile teams that include CHWs to reach remote and poor populations.

Increasing Managerial Flexibility in Public Facilities

Most UNICO countries aim to improve the supply response of public providers by increasing managerial flexibility in public clinics and hospitals, usually by allowing managers to use part of the income from demand-side payments to respond quickly to changing needs at the facility level by purchasing inputs or services outside the usually rigid rules that govern use of public funds. In the past, this flexibility only existed for funds from user fees charged by the facility; increasingly it is extended to funds from UHC programs. About 70 percent of UNICO UHC programs are attempting to improve incentives or reduce rigidities in the public sector (table 5.1).

Almost all of these programs have adopted incentives financed by allowing their public health facilities to retain part or all their income and manage cash at their own level. This gives managers of hospitals or clinics the financial autonomy to boost productivity and reward better performance. In Thailand for instance, many public hospitals have hired

TABLE 5.1
Number and Share of UHC Programs Providing Incentives for Public Health Workers

UHC programs improving incentives (or reducing rigidities) for:	Number of programs	Share of programs (%)
Hospital managers	14	52
Primary care clinic managers	13	48
Physicians	16	59
Other health workers	14	52
Any of the above	19	70

Source: UNICO studies.

more staff to respond to an increasing workload without violating the government's policy of zero growth of civil servants. UHC programs in Brazil, India, and Turkey have allowed hospitals to hire additional staff and pay extra compensation to staff working to production targets, going beyond the remuneration that standard civil service rules allow. Plan Nacer in Argentina allows public health care providers to retain the resources from the public insurer, and in some provinces these become worker incentives.

In Guatemala, mobile health teams have recruited ambulatory care/ mobile nurses when faced with doctor shortages, reflecting local needs. This response opened up a new field for nurses, and encouraged schools to develop new curricula. Doctors in the Guatemalan PEC mobile health team are eligible to receive a small incentive ($30 every three months) based on the whole team's performance in quarterly evaluations.

India's NRHM program provides financial autonomy for public health facilities, giving them additional funds to spend beyond what they receive as line-item budgets. In India's RA program, nearly a third of the insurance claim is paid as an incentive to physicians and health workers in the public health system; the program covers tertiary and some secondary procedures, and users can choose any providers from a list of those affiliated with the program. This incentive is designed to improve the responsiveness to scheme beneficiaries, because public providers compete with private providers to attract these covered patients.

The resources obtained from UHC programs are also helping gain flexibility by purchasing other goods and services. The Indian NRHM has program- or state-level initiatives where certain services are purchased from private providers, using the revenue retained in the hospital, and improving the availability and mix of services in the facility. Turkey has also introduced in its hospital reform some flexibility in equipment purchases. In Chile, Plan AUGE receives a fee-for-service payment from the public insurer, which provides additional resources to public providers that they can use for purchasing medical inputs and equipment. Likewise, in Indonesia's Jamkesmas and the Philippines Sponsored Program for Poor Families, hospital managers purchase external inputs, including diagnostic services, from third-party laboratories to augment their hospitals' capacity to provide certain services.

The UNICO case studies also show that not all incentive systems get it right at first attempt, and sometimes these incentives generate unintended consequences, which call for correction. For example:

- In China, doctors in public hospitals have overtreated patients to generate added income to their salaries.

- In Ghana, the provider-payment system is promoting curative and diagnostic services more than preventive and promotive care.

- In Vietnam, hospitals tend to focus on services that are the most profitable and not covered by the social health insurance benefit package. Part of the capitation fee is then diverted from the referring, lower-level facility to the higher-level hospital, further reducing resources for lower facilities.

While the case studies show that many countries are converging on the policies to increase flexibility and autonomy, they did not intend to provide evidence about *how well* these policies work. Further research is needed to determine the impact of these policies and the combination of incentives that will best raise health facility performance and improve effective coverage.

Increasing Participation of Private Providers

Many UNICO programs are contracting with private providers to deliver care (table 5.2). Following their countries' traditional practice, all 26 programs deliver care through public providers. What in many countries is a departure is a willingness of governments to use the UHC programs to also engage with private providers (14 programs) or philanthropic providers (12 programs) to expand capacity.

The manner in which private or philanthropic providers are engaged varies by country. Nine of them have a stated objective of expanding "choice", with the result that public and private providers offer similar services. But not all countries focus on establishing competition: many engage the private sector with very specific objectives. Some use private providers in niches where public provision is insufficient: in Guatemala,

TABLE 5.2
UHC Programs Engaging Private or Philanthropic Providers

Level of care	Countries
Primary	Brazil, China, Colombia, Georgia, Ghana, Guatemala, Jamaica, Kenya, Nigeria, South Africa, Thailand
Secondary	Chile, China, Colombia, Georgia, Ghana, India—RA, India—RSBY, Indonesia, Philippines, Thailand, Vietnam
Tertiary	Chile, China, Colombia, Georgia, Ghana, India—RA, Indonesia, Mexico, Philippines, Thailand, Vietnam

Source: UNICO studies.

for example, following the civil war large areas of the country had no public providers and nongovernmental organizations were engaged to cover the population in those areas. In Brazil, municipalities operating under the Family Health Program cannot recruit health worker teams through public channels and do so through philanthropic bodies. In some countries, only selected services are purchased from private providers: in Mexico and Vietnam for example, the UHC program uses private services only for selected tertiary services that are not offered by public providers. In Chile, because citizens are guaranteed services in the benefit package to be provided within a certain time, if this is breached, the insurer must pay for private provision.

Another use of private providers is a form of "strategic purchasing" that generates some competition, but only with low-end private services. In India's RSBY, a private insurer is selected to provide coverage to the poor population of a certain jurisdiction, this insurer must then accredit participating private and public hospitals; in practice, the best ranked or most attractive hospitals do not participate in the program, so competition is restricted to those applying and willing to provide services at the insurer's rates. In Indonesia, private hospitals must apply for a permit to operate; one of the conditions is that they cannot restrict their services to patients paying for VIP or first-class rooms—they must offer second- and third-class rooms, too. As the poor cannot afford any private rooms, third-class rooms are often underutilized, such that the hospitals are willing to accept very low rates from the UHC program to fill them.

Accrediting Health Facilities

UNICO countries are using their UHC programs to develop processes aiming to improve quality more broadly in the health system, including accrediting health facilities. Two-thirds of UNICO countries have set up such systems, under which conditions must be met for facilities to participate in the program (table 5.3 and box 5.1). Some countries are experimenting with other quality interventions (table 5.4).

The countries have introduced accreditation requirements in different ways. In Thailand, for instance, providers are contracted by the National Health Security Office (NHSO) and must meet standard conditions to join the provider network. Inspectors from that office periodically evaluate these providers on quality of care, and can cancel contracts if standards are not maintained. In other countries (see table 5.3) the Ministry of Health (MoH) or another government agency (or agencies) is responsible for a raft of measures, including monitoring service delivery, performing evaluations, following up on standards and protocols, assuring quality

TABLE 5.3
Quality Regulations and Provider Accreditation in UHC Programs

Country	Accreditation to participate	Who regulates provider participation in UHC program	Functioning penalty system
Argentina	N	N/A	N
Brazil	N	N/A	N
Chile	Y	Fonasa	Y
China	N	Private hospitals are required to be approved by local health authorities	
Colombia	Y	Provincial government	Y
Costa Rica	Y	MoH	Y
Ethiopia	N	N/A	N
Georgia	N	N/A	N
Ghana	Y	MoH	N/A
Guatemala	Y	MoH	N/A
India	Y (RA and RSBY)	MoH/Implementing government agency	Y
Indonesia	Y	N/A	N
Jamaica	N	MoH (only pharmacies are registered under the NHF)	N
Kenya	Y	MoH and HSSF funds	N/A
Kyrgyz Republic	Y	MoH	N/A
Mexico	Y	MoH	N
Nigeria	Y	Quality Assurance Department of NHIS	N
Peru	N	MoH and SUNASA (regulatory agency)	N
Philippines	Y	PhilHealth Centers (for safety, for quality, and for excellence)	N/A
South Africa	Y	MoH	N/A
Thailand	Y	MoH	Y
Tunisia	N	N/A	N
Turkey	Y	MoH	N/A
Vietnam	N for public Y for private	MoH	N

Source: UNICO studies.
Note: Y = Yes; N = No; N/A = not available.

BOX 5.1
Accreditation—A Key Condition for Getting Value for Money

Accreditation is the most commonly used external mechanism to improve quality, and governments are increasingly introducing it to regulate and provide accountability for the public health system. It is usually voluntary, sponsored by a nongovernmental organization, in which trained peer reviewers evaluate a health care organizations' compliance with standards. The focus is on organizational rather than practitioner capabilities. Performance standards for accreditation are usually developed by a consensus of health care experts, published, and regularly reviewed. Accreditation focuses on achieving optimal quality standards, unlike licensing, which focuses on compliance with minimal standards, intended to ensure public safety (Rooney and van Ostenberg 1999). Most accreditation programs offer services to both private and public sector health care organizations (Shaw 2005).

The principal component of a successful accreditation system is, per Rooney and van Ostenberg (1999), the capacity to determine a program's mission, philosophy, and key decision maker; relevant, objective, and measurable standards to achieve expected quality improvements; management of field operations, including survey supervision and training; a framework for accreditation decisions to make the process fair, valid, and credible, including a database, published performance standards, and financial viability.

Health regulatory agencies must cover the activities of all health care providers. Their most important efforts include: quality assurance at health facilities; accreditation of health care providers; and assessing standards of care as defined by the MoH. Here, the MoH has the key role of stewardship and generating norms and standards, including for quality assurance at all health facilities, clinical laboratories, and clinical practices, as well as for technologies, tools, and guidelines for PHC and hospital management, and risk and safety standards, among others. In some cases, external validation and the testing of program standards may be applied (they are not mandatory).

Accreditation systems should cover four areas: (a) supervision of health data, including audits of patient records, costing, quality of patient information, and health records; (b) supervision of standards, which include the principles and norms used as the basis for assessing hospital and health facility performance, and technology. The accreditation organization can apply these standards—focusing on quality of services—to determine if providers meet the MoH standards. This process can involve self-assessment surveys by health facilities, providing better frameworks for health care organizations to administer the quality of care throughout their systems; (c) technical support to improve quality: the accreditation agency can facilitate access to the information needed though a network of firms that specialize in this area. The support can focus on quality assurance through problem-solving, training of management and staff, improving communications between health care providers and users, accreditation and certification. An important role for the agency is to evaluate the impact of accreditation on certain indicators; and (d) protection of health rights: the agency must ensure that quality standards are followed and penalize facilities that do not comply with those that protect user rights, provide consumers with health information, and improve procedures for self-assessment and peer review by clinical providers. It is desirable that the agency also encourages universities, professional associations, and medical and nursing administrators to guarantee quality performance through continuing certification, and by promoting collection and dissemination to health care providers of national and international experience, techniques, and data.

Developing accreditation arrangements requires top-down and bottom-up strategies so as to obtain and maintain political support from all stakeholders. Initiating the process is easier than ever before, as many quality instruments (such as patient surveys, indicators, and practice guidelines) are available on the Internet and several institutes help strengthen quality and accreditation.

TABLE 5.4
Quality Provisions in Selected UNICO Countries

Country	Description of quality provisions
Ghana	NHIS conducts/approves the accreditation of providers every two years.
Guatemala	The UHC program contracts with nongovernmental organizations that must be accredited by Health Area Offices, and ultimately approved by the MoH.
Indonesia	All public and private providers must have certifications and permission to practice. Private providers must accept and enroll the poor and earmark at least 10% of their available beds for them.
Kenya	Access to HSSF funds by health facilities is subject to several basic requirements: the facility and HSSF committee have received a legal/statutory notification; the Health Facility Management Committees members have been trained; an account for HSSF is at an approved commercial bank; facilities have adequate technical and accounting staff (with at least one nurse for a dispensary and one clinical officer per health center); and facilities must prepare an annual operating plan to be approved by the district health management team.
Nigeria	All primary public and private providers are accredited by the Quality Assurance Department of NHIS using a structured checklist covering minimum requirements. Secondary public and private providers are approved by a team of NHIS staff and external experts. No provider has lost the right to participate in the program yet.
South Africa	The UHC program created accreditation procedures in which the Department of Health was tasked with inspecting every facility in every health district targeted to provide anti-retroviral treatment to ensure that it complied with accreditation requirements and provided a mix of technical and financial resources as well as training for managers and clinicians.
Turkey	The MoH has a well-developed quality assurance system for its hospitals.
Vietnam	All public providers were automatically approved to participate in SHI, but private providers needed certifications and permission, although none has lost the right to participate in recent years.

Source: UNICO studies.

control of pharmaceuticals and laboratories, conducting patient satisfaction surveys, licensing professionals, and accrediting hospitals.

Incentives play a strong role in the success of any accreditation system. While accreditation is in itself voluntary, the incentive to be part of a UHC program or a payer's network makes it nearly an imperative, depending on the size and role of the payer in the revenues (or potential revenues) of a health facility.

Without financial incentives for accreditation, health care organizations may not be motivated to join the network, as time and resources are spent attaining and maintaining accreditation. Other reasons for avoiding it include a fear of sanctions for shortcomings, loss of staff morale if accreditation is denied, misuse of performance data, and losing accreditation after obtaining it if standards are raised.

In most countries, governments find it hard to prevent the participation of public providers even if they are not accredited. Some large UHC programs—Argentina, Brazil, China, India (NHRM), and Peru—as well as small ones—Georgia and Tunisia—do not have approved or accredited providers because the regulations and quality supervision of public health care services is in theory conducted by the MoH. In some countries, public health facilities participate in the UHC programs as part of a PHC initiative and are certified by MoH agencies. In most countries, public hospitals are owned and run by various government agencies, several of which are decentralized to local governments, in which case the national MoH may not hold supervisory power. In Brazil, local governments regulate pharmacy services and accredit health facilities based on certain criteria.

Many countries have started to define accreditation standards and arrangements using a third-party agency. In Peru, a new health agency (SUNASA) was created in 2009 (and renamed SUSALUD in 2014) with the authority to accredit and penalize public and private providers, and with a remit to focus on stewardship, evaluations, and monitoring. Elsewhere, such as the Philippines, three levels of accreditation are being developed: the Center for Safety (linked to the Department of Health licensing system), the Center for Quality, and the Center of Excellence. Multiple UHC programs[1] have developed institutional arrangements to accredit providers. In Chile, AUGE runs a provider-accreditation process through the National Health Agency, but despite this mechanism most public providers, particularly hospitals, are not yet certified, although they are allowed to participate in the UHC program.

In Colombia, providers need to meet certain organizational and infrastructure standards to operate. The provincial government verifies that they meet them and issues a permit to operate, registered in a national database. Payers in the program can only contract with authorized providers, and the program contracts selectively.

In RA and RSBY in India, providers are assessed by the insurer on behalf of the government agency, and individuals enrolled in the programs can seek treatment from any of the accredited centers. India is one of the few countries where many health centers have been suspended due to failure to comply with program conditions (for example, unwillingness to participate in community-based screening camps, too few or too weak infrastructural and human resources, false claims, and charging patients for disallowed services).

The Mexican MoH (through the Dirección General de Calidad y Educación en Salud, DGCES) and the Nigerian NHIS use a checklist with standards that can be applied while supervising the health units and granting accreditation. In Mexico, this process is based on human resources and infrastructure units. However, second- and third-level care units provide services to Seguro Popular affiliates, even if they are not accredited, and then receive partial payment for services. No provider has lost the right to participate in the program.

Accreditation and regulation of quality are essential for patient safety. Most UNICO countries are introducing them, although these are still reported (see table 5.4) to be weak in design and implementation, illustrated by the fact that only few UHC programs reported actions taken against health care providers who do not comply with guidelines or were involved in malpractices. One reason may be that it is often the health ministries and other government agencies that are themselves creating and implementing these regulations in their own facilities. This lack of separation between providing and regulating care may be at the root of this problem, an area thus requiring further research.

Continuum of Care: Integrating the Health System, Strengthening Primary Care

After reviewing countries' health workforces and facilities, we now ask: How does the system perform as an integrated whole, providing a continuum of health care services to the beneficiaries over levels of care and fitting these vital pieces into the larger provision puzzle? This section provides an overview of challenges facing countries, how they are progressively pivoting toward integrated care systems, the role of PHC in that pivot, and what is needed next for the supply side to function at its best.

This last point is important because the supply side in nearly all UNICO countries is disorganized and fragmented. Some countries have a unified system of public health facilities, others a multiplicity with sometimes weak coordination among levels of care. Needless to say these systemic shortcomings affect delivery of care and, ultimately, health outcomes.

Encouragingly, UNICO countries are recognizing more and more the need for integration across the health system, aiming to give the population access to a coherent, optimally functioning network of health care providers, along the continuum of health promotion, disease prevention, diagnosis, treatment, management, rehabilitation, and palliative care (box 5.2).

Developing such an intricately organized mechanism is no easy task, as UNICO policy makers might well be the first to admit. It requires strategic reform, systematic reallocation and improved availability of resources, greater stewardship for government, tighter partnership between the private and public sectors, solid evidence bases, and adapted use of best practices. Only a few UHC programs—mainly in middle-income Argentina, Colombia, Costa Rica, Peru, Thailand, and

---

BOX 5.2

What Is Integrated Health Care and Why Can It Make a Difference?

Health care outcomes are determined not only by *technical health care factors*, but also by *how* health systems are organized, according to a growing body of evidence. How they are organized affects their capacity to provide continuous care for all life stages, to be easily accessed, to offer comprehensive, integrated, proactive care, and to create conditions where health care providers are responsible for a well-defined community or population (Macinko et al. 2007; WHO 2010; WHO and UNICEF 1978).

This is what integrated care is all about. WHO (2008) defines integrated service delivery as "the organization and management of health care services so that people get the care they need, when they need it, in ways that are user-friendly, achieve the desired results and provide value for money." Integrated care refers to the way providers function together with respect to health care services and use of resources. It also refers to "horizontal" integration (connecting similar levels of health care, for example, doctor teams in hospitals) and "vertical" integration (connecting different levels of care, from primary to tertiary).

Part of this integrative framework, "continuity of care" incorporating patients' views on practitioners' performance is often divided into three components: continuity of information (shared records); continuity across the secondary–primary interface (discharge planning from specialist to generalist care); and provider continuity (receiving services from the same professional during each visit, with value added via a developing, trusting relationship).

Integrated care generally adopts PHC as the organizing strategy because it is the main source of services within a public health system, achieving better and more equitable health outcomes at lower cost than systems oriented toward specialty care (Hsieh et al. 2013; Macinko, Starfield, and Erinosho 2009).

Turkey—have made efforts to move toward integrated care, where a vital first step has been to establish robust provision of PHC services. Examples of such integration for specialized services include Argentina, whose UHC program has several central and satellite hospitals providing care for congenital heart disease through a referral system, and Peru, with its cancer hospital network.

The importance of good PHC is well documented: initiatives to strengthen PHC, such as increasing the supply and use of PHC practitioners and improving the quality of care, are tied to better health outcomes. In low- and middle-income countries, studies have found that PHC strategies decrease infant and under-five mortality and increase life expectancy (Kruk et al. 2010; Mosquera et al. 2012).

Investing in PHC is a double header: not only an obvious choice for better health outcomes but also vital to start integrating the health system. A PHC agent is usually a beneficiary's first point of contact with the health system. Thus PHC can be a way of diagnosing and treating patients promptly and coordinating their movements smoothly through other parts of the system, provided it has a good gatekeeping and referral system. Such strong PHC coordination, with a greater hands-on role—in WHO 2010's words: "refer less, resolve more"—is the base from which to improve health outcomes and maximize human and financial resource efficiency.

It has been argued that in a PHC-based health system, the primary level of care should handle most of the health problems and should act as the communication center for the various levels of care (Mendes 2013)—referring people with conditions that require higher-level services and guaranteeing that follow-up care continues when they are discharged. Indeed, as the primary entry point to the health system, PHC facilities are best placed to establish closer links with entire communities and better understand and respond to their needs (Farmer et al. 2001).

However, the health system still needs an appropriate and reasonable mix of hospitals: hospitals are also important entities in integrated health networks—not only because they account for the largest share of the health care costs, specialized doctors, and equipment but also because their integration with secondary and PHC providers is essential to complement and complete the response to the population's health care needs. Yet most UNICO countries may have "overfocused" on hospital services, especially for services such as complicated maternity cases and many trauma and chronic disease conditions.

Still, most UNICO countries, providing PHC as well as hospital care, remain a long way from the coordinated, integrated care model. Lack of a good gatekeeping and referral system, as well as poor coordination between the primary and secondary/tertiary levels, are holding up integration (table 5.5).

Thailand is a good example of coordinated care, with an effective referral system in the public sector. The provincial health office is the main actor coordinating collaboration between the more peripheral district hospitals and the higher provincial hospitals. From provincial hospitals, seriously ill patients are further referred to regional hospitals for more intensive medical care. District hospitals are the gatekeepers, and patients cannot go directly to general or regional hospitals without a referral, except in emergencies or if they pay OOPE. The distribution of services at different levels also seems appropriate: of outpatient services, almost half (45.3 percent) are at health centers (primary care), over a third (37 percent) at district hospitals (secondary care), and 17.8 percent at provincial hospitals (tertiary care).

Integrated care in Costa Rica has also progressed, although slowly, in a context where the primary, secondary, and tertiary services are managed in a highly centralized system. Referrals and counter-referrals between health centers and the hospitals providing ambulatory and

TABLE 5.5

Integrated Care in UNICO Countries: Referrals, Integrated Networks, and Gatekeeping

Functional	Somewhat functional	Weak coordination of care (referral networks and gatekeeping)	No referrals or gatekeeping
Costa Rica (CCSS) Thailand (UCS)	Colombia	Argentina (Plan Nacer) Brazil (Sistema Único de Saúde, SUS) Chile Guatemala India Indonesia (Jamkesmas) Jamaica Kenya (Health Sector Services Fund) Kyrgyz Republic (State Social Health Insurance Program for the Poor) Tunisia (Free Medical Assistance for Poor) Vietnam (Social Health Insurance)	China Ethiopia (Health Extension Program) Georgia Ghana Mexico (Seguro Popular) Nigeria (NHIS-MDG-MCH/MSS/ MPHC) Peru (SIS) Philippines (Sponsored Program for Poor Families) Turkey Green Card (Yesil Kart)

Source: UNICO studies.

inpatient care are still weak. A slow rate of investment in modernizing and upgrading an aging hospital infrastructure impedes efficient triage of patients to the secondary or tertiary level.

Several other UNICO countries are still struggling to make progress in integrating services at different levels. In Brazil, for instance, tertiary care is mostly provided by federal hospitals (MoH and university hospitals), state governments, and some larger municipalities that also run tertiary facilities. Although some facilities follow up referrals from clinics to hospitals, most networks see few follow-ups. Brazil is an example of the difficulty in attaining integrated care in a system that has such varied sources of financing, administration, and reporting.

In Chile, AUGE has helped improve referrals because laws were enacted that defined the referral patterns. For instance, the treatment guarantee for diabetic patients involves initial consultations with a specialist to confirm the diagnosis and determine the course of treatment; this is followed by subsequent treatment at the PHC level, with occasional referrals to specialists and for hospitalization.

In Indonesia, public sector primary care services are provided by a network of *puskesmas,* which are expected to make referrals to secondary and tertiary public hospitals; if patients need more specialized care, they are referred to specialists in family medicine centers, the largest outpatient health facilities in the country. Despite the designated gatekeeping and referral roles of the *puskesmas,* they remain weak, partly because the system lacks penalties for patients who bypass the referral process and go directly to centers with higher levels of care, and usually more supplies.

Other UNICO countries have made efforts, but with limited results. In the health facilities under the Philippine Sponsored Program for Poor Families, the referral chain does not work, largely because health care services at different levels of care belong to different levels of government. Such heterogeneity—with different budgeting, administration, and reporting systems—hampers the integrated care model. In India, medical college hospitals are higher-level facilities designed for referrals. Yet the gatekeeping and referral systems are not strong and so even medical college hospitals receive many primary care cases in their outpatient facilities.

Similarly in Kenya, coordination between different levels of health care is not optimal and neither the referral networks nor the gatekeeper functions work well. The fragmented health system composed of several providers and financing institutions exacerbates the situation. Still, this is expected to change with new laws in which the country's 47 counties are being made responsible for providing primary and secondary health care delivery while the MoH will determine the overall policy and manage national referral hospitals. Under Nigeria's Midwives' Service Scheme (MSS), covering 652 PHC facilities across the country (with a greater number in the north), the country has adopted a cluster model to build a two-way referral system between primary and secondary facilities: four primary health centers are clustered around one general hospital in a local subdivision.

Conclusions and Policy Implications

The upshot to this chapter is that, while more financial resources may indeed be required for UHC, these alone are insufficient to deliver quality health care services with affordable access. Even with a well-defined and financed health coverage program with well-identified beneficiaries, a country needs a well-organized supply system.

To expand and improve their capacity to provide quality services, many UNICO programs are converging on policies. To address distribution issues of health workers, especially in remote areas, many countries are using monetary and nonmonetary incentives—including investing in their skills—to attract and retain health workers. Many are also using CHWs for outreach in rural and low-density areas. Countries are attempting to improve the effectiveness of their public providers by allowing a measure of financial autonomy to give managers of public health facilities greater flexibility to respond to changing needs. UHC services must provide quality services, and to this end many UNICO countries are introducing accreditation and tighter regulation. Finally, UNICO countries increasingly recognize the need for integration across the health system, grounded in PHC.

Policy makers implementing these moves still, however, face numerous political challenges. Among them, policies involving CHWs (which have great potential, especially when part of a larger team effort with other types of health worker) require task shifting and the definition of remuneration policies for the CHWs, and such decisions are sensitive, demanding skills in political economy. Policies to provide managers of public facilities with greater flexibility in their use of cash are often also sensitive, as they raise concerns about fiduciary risks. And while accreditation policies are now common in the UNICO countries, enforcing the requirements is often weak, especially among public providers.

Some key policy implications are:

- *Policy makers need to consider the capacity of health care provision and enhance it, as necessary, to attain their UHC objectives.* Financing is important, but a UHC program is only as good as the services it can buy, and if they are unavailable when and where needed, any effort toward UHC will be incomplete.

- *Several tools can enhance the engagement, capacity, performance, and utilization of human resources for health.* Investments in their greater effectiveness are at the heart of efforts to enhance supply, and include better performance measurement, monetary and nonmonetary incentives to reward performance, and improvements to capacity and skills. However, as incentives may have unintended consequences they may need to be revised over time, and so should be monitored closely.

- *Greater utilization of the existing health provision capacity can be a significant source of additional supply of services.* Public providers have untapped capacity, which may be used by providing greater flexibility and autonomy to the managers of public clinics and hospitals. The private sector can also be leveraged to augment service availability and countries may opt for various different roles for this sector, some of which involve choice for users while others seek complementarities in specific niches.

- *Mechanisms to ensure quality of services are integral to UHC program design.* Many countries are opting for the use of accreditation to improve quality of care. This route may offer some benefits, but it is often politically difficult to implement in both the public and private sectors. Also, more research is needed to confirm the expectation that accreditation leads to improved quality of care.

- *Gatekeeping and referral mechanisms are complex, and most countries struggle to get them right, but they should persevere.* Well-performing health systems require attention to design, implementation, and monitoring. A focus on primary care contributes to a more sustainable, accessible, and equitable health system, attaining better health outcomes at lower cost.

- *Operational knowledge needs to be strengthened.* Key areas for further research include measuring the efficiency and quality effects of providing autonomy to health facilities or managers on human resources performance; analyzing the improvement in effective coverage linked to improvements in supply; describing the functions and implementation of integrated services in health care networks, including community outreach and diagonal interventions and an assessment of why PHC clinics are bypassed; assessing the effects of mobile health units and CHWs on health outcomes in remote and poor areas; and measuring the impact on the quality of care of institutional arrangements to accredit health care providers.

Note

1. Chile, Colombia, Costa Rica, Ghana, Guatemala, Indonesia, Mexico, Nigeria, and Vietnam.

References

Farmer, P., F. Léandre, J. S. Mukherjee, M. S. Claude, P. Nevil, M. C. Smith-Fawzi, S. P. Koenig, A. Castro, M. C. Becerra, J. Sachs, A. Attaran, and J. Yong Kim. 2001. "Community-Based Approaches to HIV Treatment in Resource-Poor Settings." *The Lancet* 358 (9279): 404–9.

Hsieh, V. C., J. C. Wu, T.-N. Wu, and T. L. Chiang. 2013. "Universal Coverage for Primary Health Care Is a Wise Investment: Evidence from 102 Low- and Middle-Income Countries." *Asia-Pacific Journal of Public Health.* July. doi:10.1177/1010539513492562.

Kruk, M. E., D. Porignon, P. C. Rockers, and W. Van Lerberghe. 2010. "The Contribution of Primary Care to Health and Health Systems in Low- and Middle-income Countries: A Critical Review of Major Primary Care Initiatives." *Social Science & Medicine* 70 (6): 904–11.

Macinko, J., H. Montenegro, C. Nebot Adell, C. Etienne, and Grupo Trabaho de Atención Primaria de Salud de la Organización Panamericana de la Salud. 2007. "La renovación de la atención primaria de salud en las Américas" [Renewing Primary Health Care in the Americas]. *Revista Panamericana de Salud Pública* 21 (2–3): 73–84.

Macinko, J., B. Starfield, and T. Erinosho. 2009. "The Impact of Primary Healthcare on Population Health in Low- and Middle-Income Countries." *Journal of Ambulatory Care Management* 32 (2): 150–71.

Mendes, E. V. 2013. "Las redes de atención de salud." Organización Panamericana de la Salud, Brasilia, 549.

Mosquera, P. A., J. Hernández, R. Vega, J. Martínez, R. Labonte, D. Sanders, and M. San Sebastián. 2012. "Primary Health Care Contribution to Improve Health Outcomes in Bogotá-Colombia: A Longitudinal Ecological Analysis." *BMC Family Practice* 13: 84.

Rooney, A. L., and P. R. van Ostenberg. 1999. *Licensure, Accreditation, and Certification: Approaches to Health Services Quality.* Quality Assurance Methodology Refinement Series. Washington, DC: USAID.

Shaw, C. D. 2005. *Toolkit for Accreditation Programs: Some Issues in the Design and Redesign of External Health Care Assessment and Improvement Systems.* Dublin: International Society for Quality in Health Care.

Soucat, A., R. Scheffler, and T. Ghebreyesus, eds. 2013. *The Labor Market for Health Workers in Africa: A New Look at the Crisis.* Directions in Development. Washington, DC: World Bank.

WHO (World Health Organization). 2008. "Integrated Health Services: What and Why?" Technical Brief 1, WHO.

———. 2010. *World Health Report. Health Systems Financing: The Path to Universal Coverage.* Geneva: WHO.

WHO and UNICEF. 1978. "Declaration of Alma-Ata." International Conference on Primary Health Care, Alma-Ata, USSR, World Health Organization, Alma-Ata, September 6–12.

CHAPTER 6

Strengthening Accountability

Introduction

The topics covered in the previous four chapters might appear to constitute a comprehensive and exhaustive agenda for achieving universal coverage. In this chapter we turn our attention to a fifth topic—strengthening accountability—that in fact permeates all the others and holds an important key to achieving universal health coverage (UHC).

Various measures to strengthen accountability have been a common feature of UHC programs around the world. This suggests that in the minds of many policy makers, taking the next step toward universal coverage requires a significant departure from business as usual. In other words, it does not just entail doing more of the same—adding more (poor) people to existing coverage, more benefits to the current package, or more money and facilities to the input mix. Instead, a clear theme emerging from the Universal Health Coverage Studies Series (UNICO) is that UHC programs are often aiming to fundamentally alter the relationships between key stakeholders—levels of government, ministries, insurers, public and private facilities, personnel, and the populations they are intending to serve—through efforts to improve accountability. Indeed, in many cases entirely new (institutional) stakeholders have been established for this purpose.

Accountability matters for reasons big and small. In broad terms, it is important to ensure that a UHC program achieves its objectives, and that resources are used effectively. On a smaller scale, it can help ensure that individuals and institutions alike fulfill their responsibilities. But managing a health system is one of the most complex activities that governments take on—much more so than, for example, building a road network or paying old-age pensions (box 6.1). Thus there is ample scope for things to go wrong if one or more of the many stakeholders do not play their part.

Accountability is a commonly used but often poorly understood concept. There is no single, widely used definition, and it often seems that every commentator has a different meaning in mind. It is also hard to measure. This chapter does not aim to develop a new definition or to shed new light on the concept per se. But in order to "unpack" what is meant by the term and to organize the discussion that follows, the chapter borrows the framework for accountability as developed in the World Bank's *World Development Report* (*WDR*) *2004: Making Services Work for Poor People* (World Bank 2003). Other approaches also have their merits, but the *WDR* framework is relatively well known and is well suited to the task at hand. Only selected aspects will be highlighted here, as appropriate to highlight key characteristics of UHC programs.

Features and Key Relationships

The *WDR 2004* conceptualizes accountability as a relationship between actors that has five features: *delegation, finance, performance, information about performance*, and *enforceability* (figure 6.1). In economic jargon, it is a principal-agent relationship in which the principal *delegates* a task (or tasks) to an agent and provides *financing* for its execution. The agent then *performs* the task (well or badly), and provides *information* about what it has done. Finally, the principal holds the agent responsible for the agent's performance through various *enforcement* mechanisms, both positive (rewards) and negative (sanctions). Typically the process is then repeated.

Stronger accountability is achieved when each of these five elements is present and working well. They are mutually dependent in the sense that if one element fails, overall accountability can break down too. At the heart of these relationships is *performance*—or more specifically, eliciting good rather than bad performance. The other four elements are the essential scaffolding that helps to support good performance, and thus they will be the main focus of discussion about policies.

The *WDR* then applies this lens to three key relationships: between policy makers and providers; between the (poor) population and providers; and between the population and their policy makers (figure 6.2). Each of these broad categories has many key actors. Policy makers include technocrats and politicians, often at different levels of government (federal, state or province, municipality, etc.). Providers may be institutions such as hospitals or individual doctors, nurses, or public health workers who may practice alone or within a larger facility.

FIGURE 6.1
Five Features of Accountability

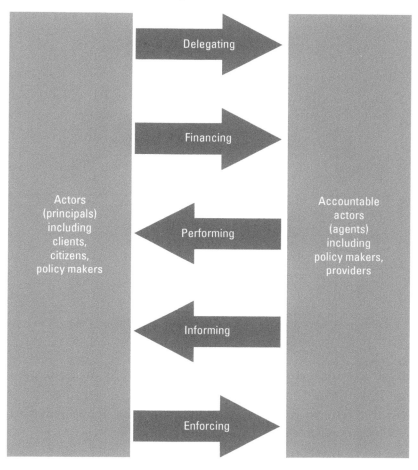

Source: World Bank 2003.

Insurance agencies could also be seen as providers. The population is considered to be "clients" when encountering providers and "citizens" when interacting with politicians and policy makers. One recurrent theme is the interaction between national and subnational policy makers in federal states, and the *WDR* accountability framework can itself be applied to the issue of decentralization.

The importance of accountability has been highlighted elsewhere. In the health systems literature, the issue of accountability has typically appeared—implicitly or explicitly—under the heading of governance and stewardship. When it was first highlighted as one of the four key functions of a health system, stewardship was defined as "setting and enforcing the rules of the game and providing strategic direction for all the

FIGURE 6.2
Key Relationships of Accountability

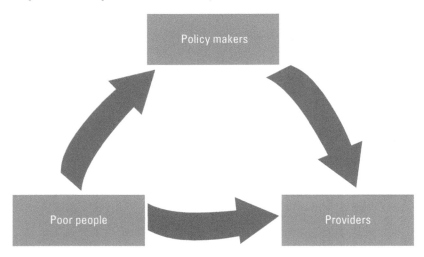

Source: World Bank 2003.

different actors involved" (WHO 2000). Over time the link between stewardship and accountability has become more explicit, as "ensuring accountability" was later identified as one of the six key stewardship functions (WHO 2007). Elsewhere, accountability in the health sector has been defined as both answerability and sanctions, and divided into financial, performance, and political accountability (Brinkerhoff 2004; Brinkerhoff and Bossert 2014).

The term "accountability" has received very little mention in much of the large literature to emerge on UHC in recent years. There are some notable exceptions, however (Rockefeller Foundation et al. 2013; WHO 2014). The discussion here aims to help close this gap by looking at how UHC programs are aiming to strengthen accountability.

Equipped with the *WDR 2004* framework depicted in the two earlier figures and based on a reading of the 26 UNICO studies, we identify four groups of policies for consideration, which form the structure of the rest of the chapter. In keeping with the main theme of this book, the discussion is organized around *how* countries are aiming to achieve UHC.

The first three groups focus almost exclusively on the "policy maker–provider" relationship depicted in figure 6.2, while the last one, empowerment, covers the other two relationships: the interaction between the population with politicians and policy makers (as citizens) and with providers (as clients).

BOX 6.1
Why Is It So Hard to Achieve Accountability in the Health Sector?

The markets for health care and health insurance are unlike most others, and therein lies the challenge of achieving accountability in this sector. There is no simple two-way relationship between buyer and seller as in a typical private good market. People (and policy makers) typically do not know when they will fall sick, and patients do not have the knowledge or expertise to diagnose and treat their illness or to judge the quality of care received. Moreover, in a state of illness they are usually not in a position to shop around for better quality or lower prices. Hospitals, laboratories, and drug companies may also have significant market power. In brief, health care markets are beset by the complicating factors of asymmetric information, moral hazard, adverse selection, third-party payers, externalities, and so on. The web of institutions commonly found in health systems is a response to this complexity, and they make it hard to achieve accountability.

Even within the realm of public services, health can be a challenging sector, for three main reasons (World Bank 2003). One is that health services, especially for curative care, are often "discretionary" in the sense that the provider must exercise significant judgment about what and how to deliver care. Contrast this with more "automated" services, such as administering a polio vaccine or making a pension payment. A second reason is that health care provision is often "transaction intensive," meaning that it requires frequent, repeated doctor–patient contact. This is especially true for managing chronic diseases. A final reason is that it can be difficult to establish "attributability" to the doctor's intervention in the event of success (or failure) of a patient's health outcome. Did they get better (or worse) because of good (or bad) medical care, or because the illness was already receding (or advancing)? There is much less ambiguity when, for example, a road is built (or not).

In brief, discretionary and transaction-intensive health care services with weak attributability are very hard to monitor, both for the patient and for the policy maker, regardless of whether they are provided in the public or the private sector. As such, they pose particular challenges for each of the five features of accountability. In other words, it can be especially difficult to delegate, finance, collect information, and enforce standards for health care services when seeking to elicit strong performance. The fact that advanced health systems around the world are also struggling to strengthen accountability highlights the reality that this is not a problem that will be solved overnight, but rather an ongoing battle in which even incremental improvements should be welcomed.

Sources: World Bank 2003.

Each group has a longer list of possible interventions. As earlier, we emphasize the *changes* to health systems during recent implementation of UHC programs that expanded coverage for the poor. The concluding section discusses which policies seem to be working well, and where the challenges appear to loom larger, implying a need for more work in order to strengthen their contribution to UHC programs.

Delegating—Toward Arm's-Length Relationships and Explicit Responsibilities

The first feature of an accountable relationship among actors in the *WDR* framework is *delegation*, which is defined as an "explicit or implicit understanding that a service will be supplied." Put simply, delegation addresses the question "what is to be done, and by whom?" It should be apparent that without an adequate answer to this question, accountability and thus program outcomes are likely to suffer.

Two key themes emerge from the UNICO studies in the context of delegation. The first is a trend toward more arm's-length relationships between the actor who delegates the task and the one who is responsible for carrying it out. This is especially true in the case of purchasers and providers. In other words, there is a marked shift away from integrated public financing and delivery of health care under UHC schemes. The second theme is that responsibilities are increasingly being made more explicit when the task is delegated. This is apparent in settings as varied as the definition of benefit packages and central–subnational relations in federal states.

Trend toward More Arm's-Length Relationships

The introduction of more arm's-length relationships is particularly apparent in the context of the purchasing and provision of health care services, reflecting a move toward a purchaser–provider split and thus a departure from the classic model of a Ministry of Health (MoH) allocating inputs to public facilities that are essentially budgetary units of the ministry itself (see table 6.1). Many countries have, however, made only a partial shift, with traditional MoH-run models still prominent.

UHC programs manage these relationships in many ways, such as creating a separate purchasing agency outside the MoH to contract with public providers, engaging private insurers or providers, and granting more autonomy to public providers, especially hospitals. These reforms create more space between the purchasing agent and the health care provider.

Many countries have created new agencies, charging them with purchasing care from public (and sometimes private) providers. In Thailand for example, the National Health Security Office was created to serve as an autonomous state agency with responsibility for contracting and purchasing. In the Kyrgyz Republic, the MHIF was created to be the single purchaser under UHC. Jamaica established the National Health Fund as a statutory entity covering among other things pharmaceuticals provided

TABLE 6.1
Purchaser-Provider Split in UHC Schemes

Purchaser–provider split?	Countries
Yes	Argentina, Ghana, Philippines, Thailand, Georgia,[a] Indonesia,[b] Chile, China, Colombia, Guatemala, Jamaica, Kenya,[c] South Africa, Turkey, Vietnam, Nigeria, Peru, Kyrgyz Republic, India (RSBY), India (RA)
No	Brazil, Costa Rica, India (NRHM),[d] Mexico, Tunisia

Source: UNICO studies.
a. Except for some HMOs.
b. Split introduced in 2014.
c. Separate governance for HSSF.
d. Autonomy in fund management.

at public and private facilities. In India, RSBY created State Nodal Agencies at state level to serve as the main supervisory and implementing agency responsible for contracting and monitoring insurance companies. Under the NRHM program, State Health Societies are autonomous agencies created to implement the program, and mirrored at district level by District Health Societies. In the Philippines and Vietnam, coverage for the poor was implemented by incorporating the existing social insurance agencies (PhilHealth and VSS) that already purchased health care services for formal sector workers.

In some of the studies, the *absence* of a purchaser–provider split is cited as one of the key challenges for implementing a UHC—as with Seguro Popular in Mexico. It also held true in Indonesia, but the Jamkesmas insurance program was transferred out of the MoH into a single, not-for-profit social insurance administrator in early 2014, thus joining the trend.

An alternative approach is to fully outsource the purchasing of health care to the private sector. In Colombia, Georgia, and India (both the national RSBY program and some state-level insurance programs), policy makers contracted private insurance companies to purchase health care services—including from public providers—under the UHC schemes. Nigeria's Ondo State uses health maintenance organizations (HMOs) as part of its health insurance model. The experiences in these countries have been mixed, but the motivation in all cases was greater confidence in the purchasing capacities of private sector actors.

The decision to allow public purchasing agencies to begin contracting private providers is de facto another way to implement a greater purchaser–provider split. A significant feature of UHC schemes in, for example, Chile, India, Indonesia, the Philippines, and Thailand was to begin contracting with private providers. Georgia's flagship MIP for the poor was implemented in parallel with privatization of nearly all health care providers in the country. This logic has also been extended to individual health personnel. A key element of India's NRHM program, for example, was that it started to contract accredited social health activist workers and thereby sidestep the pitfalls of civil service hiring. Similar steps to avoid the strictures of civil service employment were undertaken in Brazil and Turkey. In Guatemala, a key feature of the PEC has been to contract with nongovernmental organizations for service delivery of a basic health package. The pros and cons of circumventing weak public systems, instead of trying to fix them, deserve careful consideration but are beyond the scope of this chapter. In total, more than half the UHC programs include private providers at one or more level of care. And unlike the rhetoric of decades past, this shift does not appear to represent a step toward, or belief in, wholesale marketization of the health sector, but rather a more modest step toward greater pluralism.

Establishing an arm's-length relationship between the purchasers and providers does not have to be as blunt as a shift to private insurance and providers. Many UHC schemes are also associated with granting more autonomy to public sector providers. Autonomy has been defined as the extent of the "decision rights" that facilities have over the many and varied aspects of producing health care services. These include decisions over labor and capital inputs, fund management, output level and mix, among others (Preker and Harding 2003). Provider autonomy is particularly important in the hospital setting, where decision making is more complex. The basic rationale is to "let the managers manage."

For example, a key feature of India's NRHM program is that it introduced financial autonomy for public health facilities, allowing them to retain and flexibly spend funds instead of imposing strict line-item budgets. This was unprecedented in India's public financial management system. Provider autonomy was also granted to facilities receiving resources under Argentina's Plan Nacer program. In Kenya's UHC program, there is a significant role for community committees in determining how funds are spent. The Kyrgyz Republic introduced some limited financial and managerial autonomy to providers. Turkey introduced hospital autonomy that allowed greater flexibility for hiring staff and buying equipment. In Colombia, public providers were transformed into independent public sector enterprises. A lack of autonomy was cited as a key challenge facing Indonesia's and the Philippines' UHC schemes.

However, autonomy without oversight can prove harmful: in Vietnam, the case study identifies problems tied to enterprising hospitals taking advantage of their autonomy to flout the rules. The substantial autonomy of hospitals in China has also posed a challenge, especially in pharmaceutical sales. The transition toward more arm's-length relationships arguably makes information flows and citizen empowerment even more important (see below).

What does the literature say about these reforms? One of the oldest debates in health policy is between the so-called "Beveridge" National Health System and "Bismarck" Social Health Insurance models, but it has long been noted that this distinction is outmoded, as hybrid models predominate in most advanced health systems. It is notable that "separating the policy maker from the provider" is offered as a key option for increasing accountability in *WDR 2004*. But it has been argued that the evidence that a purchaser-provider split produces better outcomes is in fact quite thin (Wagstaff 2010). This may be partly because such reforms are difficult to rigorously evaluate. It is also true, however, that integrated public delivery models are now in the minority among advanced health systems (for example, across Organisation for Economic Co-operation and Development [OECD] countries), and in this respect many UHC programs represent a step in the same direction.

The trend to more arm's-length relationships may not be well suited to all countries seeking to make progress toward UHC. Lower-income countries, in particular, may not have adequate capacity to successfully implement these arrangements. The contracting procedures necessitated by a purchaser-provider split, for example, are more complex than what is needed under integrated public sector financing and delivery. Moreover, some middle-income countries, such as Malaysia and Sri Lanka, have had well-performing health systems for decades without any such split. Still, the trend among UHC programs is to pursue this avenue for reform.

Shift toward More Explicit Roles and Responsibilities at Task Delegation

The second major theme is a shift toward more explicit identification of roles and responsibilities, notably in two domains: the definition of the benefit package, and national–subnational relations. In both cases the rationale is simple enough: clearer expectations and responsibilities will lead to greater accountability.

In the benefit package definition, a key example comes from Chile, where the national health fund (Fonasa) did not have an explicit benefit package before the AUGE program was introduced in 2005, leading to service rationing, including through waiting lines and outright denial of care. A central goal of AUGE was to define an explicit package for Fonasa beneficiaries and to achieve greater equality in access to care between this group and the (richer) Isapres beneficiaries. The lack of a national benefit package had previously been seen as a key weakness that led to abuses and inequalities, and thus a core objective of AUGE was to bridge this gap. In fact AUGE went beyond making the benefit package explicit, by providing guarantees for waiting times, clinical pathways, and drug availability.

Other countries that have sought to achieve greater clarity in the benefit package through the UHC program include Argentina, Brazil, Georgia, India, the Kyrgyz Republic, Mexico, and Thailand. Twenty-one countries have explicit packages; three do not—Costa Rica, India (NRHM), and Tunisia (chapter 3).

The notion that clearly defining a benefit package can improve accountability and transparency is also prominent in deliberations about the future of the United Kingdom's National Health Service, which does not do so (Rumbold, Alakeson, and Smith 2012). An explicit package can strengthen accountability both by ensuring that covered services are in fact provided as well as by drawing boundaries to clarify which services are not covered (chapter 3). But doubts have been raised as to how far this logic actually applies in the real world, especially for services where scope for implicit rationing remains, such as elective surgery. Robust mechanisms for redress are also required. Improved accountability may also come at the expense of other goals. A clear benefit package may also empower pressure groups who want the package expanded (compromising sustainability), and possibly abet the emergence of private insurance packages (posing a threat to equity).

Greater clarity in the delegation of responsibilities is a feature of several UHC schemes in federal states. In many countries health is decentralized and is becoming more so (Kenya is a recent example). Most of these lower government levels are elected, and so the decentralization is political as well as administrative. In principle, decentralization can strengthen the accountability between policy makers and the citizens they serve. Local governments are potentially more accountable to local demands, as well as being in a better position to perform a range of tasks, from identifying the poor to monitoring provider performance. But decentralization also poses challenges such as capacity constraints at lower levels and greater risk of inequality due to uneven implementation across a country.

The concept of accountability is very much relevant to the principal–agent relationship between national and subnational governments. Indeed, the *WDR 2004* accountability framework has been applied to the issue of decentralization to highlight its importance in this context (Devarajan, Khemani, and Shah 2007). The implication is that the central government in a federal state must itself pay careful attention to each of the five features of accountability in their relationship with lower levels of state. In delegation, beyond providing clarity on roles and responsibilities this has meant offering wide latitude for subnational units to run the programs themselves. In this sense there is a parallel with the rationale for extending provider autonomy.

Argentina offers a good example of clear-cut delegation of responsibilities to subnational level. Under Plan Nacer, the relationship between the national and provincial MoHs is governed by legally binding management agreements. These define each party's responsibilities under an "umbrella agreement." Each year they negotiate the targets for enrollment and tracers, work programs, and resource requirements, which are included in a contract called the Annual Performance Agreement. (There is also a unique financing arrangement between the national and provincial governments, discussed in the next section.) The explicit nature of these agreements is a fundamental reason behind Plan Nacer's strong track record.

Other examples include Brazil and China. Brazil has explicit agreements between levels of government (including municipalities, which are key in health care delivery). These accords outline responsibilities, program indicators, and targets. China has opted for a mixed approach. The national government provides clear and ambitious targets to local authorities for enrollment, supported by central financing. But other aspects of implementation come under a strategy to "define broad objectives and enforce minimum requirements," allowing local authorities substantial scope for innovation and piloting.

The case study in which the interplay between national and subnational governments has been perhaps the most problematic is the Philippines. The health insurer, PhilHealth, and local government units (LGUs) have a multilayered relationship. PhilHealth relies on LGUs to enroll members but is also expected to hold them accountable for service delivery. This creates problems. Further, the case study notes that "since decentralization, the DOH (Department of Health) has had a difficult time obtaining timely access to data from providers, both LGU and private. This has made it difficult for DOH to regularly track program implementation." (These difficulties are revisited in the financing section.) Another example of problematic national–subnational relations is Peru, mainly because the shift to decentralization in 2004–05 failed to define the relationship between the levels of government.

The experiences of UHC programs in a context of decentralization reflect broader challenges in this area. A desire for national standard-setting (for example, with respect to eligibility criteria, benefit packages, accreditation, and service delivery) as a way to address inter-regional inequality would suggest that more central control of UHC programs is preferable. Similarly, economies of scale in certain aspects of program delivery (for example, the need for only one health technology agency or the advantages of centralized procurement) and possible capacity constraints at lower levels of government also point to the benefits of a stronger national footprint. But the need to reap the benefits of local knowledge and ownership and to respond to heterogeneity of demand for services across regions seems to dictate the opposite (greater local control). Measures to improve accountability are mutually dependent, with failure in one domain likely to undermine prospects in another, and nowhere is this more true than in the interaction between accountability's delegation and financing measures, to which we now turn.

Financing—Paying for Outputs and Results Instead of Inputs

The second of the five features is *finance*, and here we are specifically interested in the implications of finance (which has been discussed extensively in earlier chapters) for accountability. The central theme that emerges is that many UHC programs represent a marked shift from input-based financing to more output- and results-based approaches, as evident in three domains: most classically, in the payment of providers by purchasers; as a per capita premium-based incentive to encourage enrollment of the targeted population by those responsible for this task; and in the transfer of resources from central to subnational authorities. In some countries there is overlap between the second and third domains. These changes are rarely, however, wholesale reforms to the entire payment system, and are typically introduced alongside existing input-based financing methods.

Output-based payments in the realm of purchasing care take several different forms. These include capitation-based primary care (especially when coupled with provider choice), fee-for-service methods, and case-based payments such as DRGs. Most ambitiously, some include pay-for-performance linked to health outcomes instead of activity volumes. All these methods represent a shift from input-based approaches such as paying on the basis of salaries, bed capacity, historical line-item budgets, or simple global budgeting.

Output-based payment mechanisms are often proposed to improve accountability due to the signal they send to providers: that the services they provide to patients are their core responsibility and therefore the basis on which they will be paid. They have the potential to better align financing with the health care-seeking behavior of the population, and thus help to strengthen incentives to provide the necessary medical services to patients and to be responsive to their needs. In its absence, providers are more likely to neglect their responsibilities.

There are plenty of caveats here, of course: in particular, payment mechanisms need to be mindful of efficiency considerations, and thus open-ended, retrospective fee-for-service reimbursement of all costs is not viable. Such mechanisms may also require accompanying reforms to civil service and public financial management arrangements, and they are certainly more complex to administer. Nonetheless, output-based payments offer a potentially important piece of the puzzle when accountability is weak in an input-based payment model.

Twenty countries have adopted output-based payment methods—the only exceptions are Costa Rica, India (NRHM), Mexico, and South Africa. The Kyrgyz Republic replaced Soviet line item–based financing with population-based (for primary care) and output-based (for hospitals) reimbursements. Thailand introduced DRGs (with a global budget cap) for hospital payment. Indonesia also uses DRGs for hospitals. India's RSBY program uses output-based payments, in contrast to the supply-side NRHM model, although the latter introduced entirely performance-based pay for its (contracted) accredited social health activist workers, a novel approach for the Indian public sector. In 2013 Turkey introduced an ambitious pay-for-performance model for addressing NCDs (and other services) at primary care level, in a system that already combined capitation with substantial flexibility for patients to change their provider of choice. Under Plan Nacer, Argentina started to pay providers on a fee-for-service basis, switching from inputs. In contrast, the continued use of input-based payment by Mexico's Seguro Popular is one of the key weaknesses of an otherwise successful program, according to the case study.

Provider payment (as presented here) and provider autonomy (previous section) work best when implemented hand in hand, as creating payment-based incentives without the decision-making power to act on them is unlikely to succeed. Several UNICO studies identify tensions between approaches to payment and autonomy. In the Philippines, hospitals owned by LGUs could submit claims for services to PhilHealth, but because they were not allowed to retain income (for lack of autonomy) the money would go to the LGU instead of the hospital itself, and the LGU would then distribute funds based on historical line items. As the case study notes, "while PhilHealth payment mechanisms follow the principle that money follows the patient, in the absence of autonomy, hospitals are not able to use the funds to improve performance." A similar problem was encountered when PhilHealth tried to introduce advance payments to address cash flow problems, as the LGU hospitals did not have the autonomy to manage the funds. Addressing hospital autonomy is now prominent on the country's reform agenda. Indonesia had similar problems due to inconsistency between its payment method and a lack of autonomy at primary care level.

The idea that output-based payments are necessary to improve provider performance reflects a certain view of what motivates health workers. It emphasizes "extrinsic" motivation—derived from financial reimbursement or other rewards such as professional advancement—as opposed to "intrinsic" motivation based on a desire to help others or fulfill professional norms (Leonard, Serneels, and Brock 2013). While there is growing evidence from RBF schemes that extrinsic incentives in the form of performance-based pay can change health workers' behavior, and these findings have captured much attention in policy debates, pecuniary self-interest is not the only thing that motivates health workers. Interventions aimed at boosting intrinsic motivation, such as professional recognition and peer review, can also have a significant positive effect on the quality of health care services (Peabody et al. 2006). And some of the most successful health systems in middle-income countries like Malaysia and Sri Lanka do not rely on output-based financing at all (though they both have extensive dual practice—that is, a doctor can work in both the public and the private sector). It is also unclear how extrinsic and intrinsic motivation interact with each other—for example, extrinsic incentives may result in "crowding out" by discouraging the intrinsically motivated from joining the profession (Leonard, Serneels, and Brock 2013). In brief, it would seem that the superiority of output-based provider payment is open to debate.

Output-based payments are not limited to the purchaser-provider relationship. In several countries they are also used to transfer resources from the central to subnational government. Notably, a central feature of Plan Nacer is that transfers from the national government to provinces are made in two installments: the first, 60 percent of the total, is linked to the enrollment of beneficiaries, the second, 40 percent, to verification that targets for 10 health indicators (tracers) have been achieved. Thus, the payment mechanism incentivizes both enrollment and service delivery.

In Brazil, federal transfers to municipalities have two components, a fixed per-capita amount and a variable amount linked to achieving program targets as laid out in the intergovernmental agreement on primary care. In Mexico, before UHC reform, transfers from the center to the states were based on infrastructure and personnel, but Seguro Popular replaced this approach with transfers of actuarially calculated premiums for each beneficiary, which helped to rapidly expand coverage. Other options have been used to help motivate subnational governments via fiscal transfers, including earmarking, lump-sum grants, capitation, and matching grants.

Some federal-state financing arrangements have not been as successful. In the Philippines, LGUs were supposed to pay for care in the early years of the program, but since 2012 this has been replaced with national government support. Vietnam has a capitation-based transfer to the subnational level, but because it is based on historical utilization, it only serves to reinforce inequalities between rich and poor. In Mexico, despite the success of Seguro Popular in providing incentives to states to enroll beneficiaries, it did not similarly motivate service delivery by modifying the provider-payment method.

Output-based payments are also sometimes implemented with contracted partners such as private insurers. In India, under RSBY, insurers have an incentive to enroll as many eligible families as possible because their premium-based income is derived from the number of cards issued. In Georgia, the number of beneficiaries was set by government, but insurers competed for the vouchers issued to the poor. (However, this led to abuses due to a lack of adequate monitoring and oversight, and the system was later changed). Many of the UHC programs provided a financial incentive to the entity responsible for enrollment.

The experiences of UHC programs in the domain of output-based financing are generally reported positively in the case studies, even if the superiority of this approach is not proven. An additional advantage of this approach is that it typically generates more information and data about service delivery (as that is the basis on which payments are made) than input-based approaches.

Information and Enforcement—Collecting More Data, but Not Always Making Use of It

The fourth and fifth features of an accountable relationship as proposed in the introduction are the provision of *information* about performance and *enforcement*. The *WDR 2004* framework refers to information as "obtaining relevant information and evaluating performance against expectations and formal or informal norms." It defines enforcement as "being able to impose sanctions for inappropriate performance or provide rewards when performance is appropriate." This section begins by addressing these issues at the level of day-to-day implementation, and then considers what they mean for accountability with regard to performance of a UHC program as a whole.

Strong information flows are essential for monitoring UHC program implementation, ensuring compliance with established rules and regulations, preventing fraud, and making decisions about rewards and sanctions (if these are administered). It is also important for what might be termed "operational research" or continuous performance improvement. Almost any objective, not least quality and efficiency, will ultimately be achieved as much through micro implementation as through macro reform. Facility-level and service-specific indicators are needed to better understand the distribution of performance across all providers in the health system. For example, which hospitals have the best outcomes in case of stroke, or the most readmissions? Which doctors order the most tests or prescribe the most antibiotics? Access to this type of information can be used to work toward overall system improvement.

Nearly every UNICO study cites significant data collection efforts through health management information systems (HMIS) and general information technology (IT) systems (table 6.2 shows some characteristics). At its best, the information collected plays a pivotal role in program implementation. This is the case, for instance, of the performance indicators measured in Argentina and Brazil's programs that are used to determine fiscal transfers (chapter 4). But in many cases, availability and use of program information falls well short of this ideal.

A few countries are aiming to signal the importance of data reporting by directly incentivizing information provision. For example, Thailand provides bonuses to facilities for reporting data on time and in full, in

TABLE 6.2
Information Systems (Number of UHC Programs with Each Characteristic)

Characteristic	Yes	No
System that tracks use of health care by enrollees	22	4
Information on quality reporting (infection rates, readmission rates, outcome information)	14	12
Information on provider output/volume information, case mix	19	7
Information on grievance redress status	12	14
Program is required to specifically report on progress toward specific goals	10	8
Any instances of policy change due to a higher level authority reviewing such information from the program?	7	9
Public information available, whether passively or actively	21	4
Legal framework for disclosure of information by program on demand by external entities (such as right to information law)	14	5
Regular system of on-site inspection or field visits exists	16	11
Clear guidelines and reporting formats whereby findings are systematically reported	10	7

Source: UNICO studies.
Note: Numbers do not always add up to 26 due to missing information.

part because this information is essential for calculating relative DRG weights. In Brazil, municipalities must populate the HMIS with data; failure to do so can lead to a suspension of transfers from national government.

However, a weak information environment, or minimal use of data or monitoring and evaluation, is identified in multiple case studies, including Brazil (despite some successes), China, Georgia, Indonesia, Jamaica, Mexico, Nigeria, the Philippines, Tunisia, Turkey, and Vietnam. The following from the Philippines case study may be taken as indicative of the challenges facing many countries: "although DOH hospitals are expected to submit hospital reports to the DOH, the information is sometimes incomplete and missing key information. The DOH does not impose sanctions on hospitals that do not submit reports or that submit incomplete reports. The last consolidated hospital report for DOH hospitals was produced in 2004."

Various efforts are aimed at strengthening accountability through enforcement. Audits, both financial and technical, are common across many UHC programs. Third-party verification is an important aspect of results-based financing schemes. Chile and the Kyrgyz Republic have invested in new IT systems to help with compliance monitoring. In Argentina, Plan Nacer disincentivizes enrollment of ineligible individuals (a problem in many countries) because compliance with enrollment requirements is audited both internally and externally, and there are monetary penalties for provinces when individuals who do not meet eligibility criteria are enrolled.

But enforcement has often fallen short. Vietnam has a rule prohibiting balance billing by hospitals (resulting in high out-of-pocket expenditure [OOPE] by patients), but it is not enforced and so the practice continues. In the Philippines, without compliance monitoring, the incentives were not strong enough for providers to comply with the rules and regulations, though since 2006 PhilHealth has developed a "balanced scorecard" to tackle this.

Numerous barriers block progress on using information. Ministries of health and health insurance agencies often lack skilled professionals who can undertake the operational research on the abundant data they have collected. Health care management and health economics are new fields of study in low- and middle-income countries. Collecting and using information from key stakeholders has proven especially hard in countries with private insurance companies. In Georgia and India (RSBY), human resource constraints in the area of claims management is cited as a key challenge. In Colombia, government investigations revealed widespread fraud by insurance companies as well as some municipalities.

A more fundamental question related to the collection and use of information is whether anyone knows if a UHC program is working or not. That is, are there any systematic efforts to monitor and evaluate the impact on health outcomes, financial protection, and other key indicators? Usually, the answer is "no." Fewer than half the UHC programs have regular reporting on health outcomes. The systematic collection of data to measure financial protection and equity is even less common. As discussed in appendix C, rigorous impact evaluations of UHC programs are also quite rare. (Where they do exist, they tend to analyze overall program performance and not the impact of individual components). Thus, somewhat paradoxically given the enormous effort poured into setting up and implementing UHC programs around the world, surprisingly little is known about whether they are having a positive impact on the lives of their intended beneficiaries.

Why is there so little effort to monitor and evaluate UHC programs vis-à-vis their major objectives? In part it is a symptom of the broader problem of weak stewardship, including the absence of a culture of "evidence-based policy making." There is also weak analytical capacity to process and analyze data at the central level (especially more complex indicators such as financial protection), and often a lack of administrative staff at the provider level. There may also be weak incentives for providers to report data to central authorities, especially if payment is not linked to outputs. Politicians may not be interested if a positive impact is only likely to materialize after their current tenure or mandate is over. All this adds up to little accountability or data with which to monitor program performance.

A further possible explanation is political economy. Of course, many people may not actually want to know. A fear of information that might uncover shortcomings—whether it is poor performance or corruption, among policy makers or providers—could be a reason. Alternatively, UHC advocates may decide to neglect knowledge creation because credible estimates of program impact may undermine their ability to mobilize political and budgetary support. This is a broader challenge related to the political economy of monitoring and evaluation in general (Pritchett 2002).

Whatever the reason, the mindset has to be changed. A UHC monitoring framework has been proposed at global level, which identifies key indicators to measure progress toward UHC, including health and financial protection (World Bank and WHO 2014). This would require significant support to implement at the country level. There is also a risk that such a framework—and the implied cross-country benchmarking—would generate fears and pressures among policy makers. These political economy challenges will have to be surmounted.

Empowerment—Strengthening Citizen Voice and Client Power

The previous three sets of policies have focused largely on the relationship between politicians and policy makers on one hand and providers on the other. This final section shifts to the other two accountability relationships shown in figure 6.2: between the population and politicians (as citizen voice) and between the population and providers (as client power). In the quest for better service delivery, these are called the long and short routes of accountability, respectively, in the *WDR 2004* framework.

The mere presence of a UHC scheme reflects, for many countries, a recent improvement in the responsiveness of the government to population wishes for expanded coverage—a measure of success along the long route of accountability. In Thailand and Turkey, major reforms were undertaken in the early 2000s soon after new governments took office with a commitment to rural voters instead of urban elites. In Brazil and Peru, the UHC initiative followed soon after a return to democracy. China put greater focus on reforming the health sector in the wake of the SARS epidemic, which brought to the forefront citizen concerns about health system effectiveness. Sri Lanka launched universal coverage in the 1930s soon after universal suffrage was introduced.

But the role of citizen voice does not end with the launch of a UHC program. There is ample scope for social accountability interventions (also sometimes called demand-side governance or empowerment) to help improve effectiveness, for which citizens ideally need two tools: access to information and the opportunity to use the information and transform it into action (Ringold et al. 2012).

On the information side, interventions include access-to-information legislation, information campaigns, report cards (which provide information about service performance to citizens), scorecards (surveys of citizen satisfaction with services followed up by a facilitated meeting with providers and beneficiaries), and social audits (participatory audits in which the community compares expenditures with actual services delivered). But to transform it into action, citizens need grievance-redress mechanisms, or a channel for complaints and giving feedback. These may be in government agencies, such as the MoH, or in independent bodies. A last resort is an effective court system.

The case studies provide some examples of such steps for enhanced social accountability. One of the most common is the legislative angle, including "right to health" constitutional mandates (especially prominent in Latin America, including Argentina, Chile, and Colombia, where there was a landmark ruling in 2008) and patient rights legislation. This "judicialization" of the right to health offers significant promise as a means to strengthen accountability (Iunes, Cubillos-Turriago, and Escobar 2012). However, it also poses a risk to health system efficiency due to the prospect of rapid adoption of new health care technologies, and may have an impact on equity because access to justice, like health, often favors the rich. A comprehensive survey on the right to health has been undertaken globally (Backman et al. 2008). This issue is part of a broader shift toward judicial enforcement of social and economic rights (Gauri and Brinks 2008).

Making the benefit package explicit—common in many countries—is also a form of empowering beneficiaries to understand their rights and to reduce the chances of informal payments or denial of access to specific services. Both Chile and Mexico accompanied this with outreach to program recipients through public information campaigns. In Argentina, beneficiary demand for services was incentivized through such campaigns that informed people of their rights, services available, as well as information about child health monitoring, contributing to an ethos of social accountability.

But whether an explicit benefit package translates into better public knowledge is open to debate. A study in the early years of Chile's AUGE program found that a large share of respondents were not familiar with the package (World Bank 2008). The same was true in Georgia (Bauhoff, Hotchkiss, and Smith 2010). Actual citizen participation in the definition of benefit packages in UHC programs has been minimal. On a more positive note, informal payments are not reported to be a major issue in most UHC programs (see chapter 4). Since these are often a symptom of poor accountability, this is a welcome pattern.

Indonesia, the Kyrgyz Republic, and Turkey have introduced complaints hotlines. Georgia established a mediation service for settling disputes between private insurers and MIP beneficiaries. India's extensive use of IT, including biometric smart cards, has strong potential to help citizens who might otherwise be denied care. Some countries, such as Vietnam, offered little evidence of social accountability measures to support UHC (table 6.3).

In Kenya, the introduction of the HSSF to directly provide resources to facilities was accompanied by the creation of Health Facility Management Committees (HFMCs), which aim to ensure community participation and oversight in the use of funds. In essence, communities, represented by HFMCs, manage the funds received and prioritize their use based on community-expressed needs. This has been successful, although the complaint redress mechanisms that give voice to citizens remain weak and lack efficiency and transparency.

TABLE 6.3
Opportunities for Citizen Voice/Client Power (Number of Programs)

Characteristic	Yes	No
Information on grievance and redressal status	12	14
Public information available, whether passively or actively	21	4
Legal framework for disclosure of information by program on demand by external entities (such as a right to information law)	14	5
Are rules regulating access to the benefit package widely publicized?	19	7
Is it clear to which public official or agency patients should go if they want to file a complaint about access or quality of the services?	21	4
Does the UHC program have a patient advocate or ombudsman function?	7	17

Source: UNICO studies.
Note: Numbers do not always add up to 26 due to missing information.

Lastly, greater patient choice of provider, including through contracting the private sector, can provide citizens with an option to "vote with their feet" in favor of certain providers over others, which can help reinforce a message of accountability. This has happened in, for example, India, Indonesia, the Philippines, Thailand, and Turkey.

But evidence on the effectiveness of all these program initiatives is mixed (Ringold et al. 2012). Among the UHC measures, for example, Indonesia's complaints mechanism was reportedly not working well due to low levels of socialization and awareness of benefits. Georgia's experiment with insurer choice did not go well (a large share of beneficiaries were not even aware of having a choice) and was abandoned in favor of an alternative approach.

Much is yet to be learned, and notably, as a way to improve services, approaches to enhance the demand-side through social accountability are far less developed and discussed than interventions on the provider side, such as results-based financing. There is ongoing work to better understand the contextual factors underlying effective social accountability mechanisms (World Bank 2014). It is an area for more operational research going forward.

Conclusions

The UHC programs across the 24 countries do much more than add people, services, or money to a health system. Instead they aim to fundamentally change the way that stakeholders interact, alongside the (implicit or explicit) objective of strengthening accountability. In *delegation*, their efforts have resulted in more arm's-length relationships; *finance* has seen a partial shift toward greater reliance on output-based financing; UHC programs are making strenuous data collection efforts in *information*—but less so on using it for *enforcement;* and many programs have interventions for greater client voice.

The vast majority of case studies viewed the *delegation* and *finance* measures positively, and addressing their absence was cited as a key reform imperative in others, especially in middle-income countries, where the capacity to implement these contractual arrangements is usually stronger. It is less clear, however, that low-income countries should hasten to adopt the same measures, despite some examples of success. But as many countries are introducing demand-side financing in parallel with traditional supply-side financing, the implications of this dual-track approach warrant closer attention.

There is little definitive, rigorous evidence that the reforms in *delegation* and *finance* are the right ones, but perhaps that is true of most health system reform topics. Policies such as a purchaser-provider split and output-based payments are often championed, but they are not found in the government health systems of historically successful middle-income countries such as Malaysia and Sri Lanka. While definitive evidence on what is working may be elusive, these measures for better accountability do bring the health systems covered in the case studies closer in line with those in high-income countries. For example, a shift toward hospital autonomy has been observed across advanced European health systems in recent years (Chevalier, Garel, and Levitan 2009; Saltman, Duran, and Dubois 2011). Few OECD health systems rely on input-based financing of health care, and almost none do so at the hospital level (Paris, Devaux, and Wei 2010).

The experience of UHC programs in the areas of *information* and *enforcement,* and *empowering citizens* is mixed. Many countries are either struggling (information) or have only made tentative measures (citizen voice/client power). In all countries, questions about how to establish a culture of "evidence-based policy making" that draws on the new information flows by applying well-developed expertise in monitoring and evaluation, and how to empower citizens to hold politicians, policy makers, and providers accountable for UHC implementation, also remain unanswered.

Lastly, very few UHC programs were found to be systematically measuring program impact on key objectives such as better health outcomes and financial protection, and thus no one was being held accountable for program success or failure. The reasons for this are not fully clear—whether it is a capacity constraint, political economy, or something else—but it is clearly an issue that warrants urgent attention. Without it, the accountability agenda for UHC will remain very incomplete.

The key implication of these findings for UHC practitioners (and those who aim to support them) is that to strengthen accountability, greater effort is needed in information and empowerment. In particular, more operational research is clearly needed, for example, to help identify who has been successful at establishing effective monitoring systems; how to implement IT reforms; how to create stakeholder support for strong information flows; how and where to create analytical capacity for monitoring UHC programs; and how best to empower patients and citizens to hold providers and politicians accountable. These more specific questions have arguably been neglected in policy discussions on UHC, which have instead focused on "macro-issues" such as whether to adopt an insurance model or not. Most countries pursuing UHC reforms have already made a decision on the macro topics, and thus it is on the more specific issues that they need greater assistance in charting a path forward.

References

Backman, G., P. Hunt, R. Khosla, C. Jaramillo-Strouss, B. M. Fikre, C. Rumble, D. Pevalin, D. A. Páez, M. A. Pineda, A. Frisancho, D. Tarco, M. Motlagh, D. Farcasanu, and C. Vladescu. 2008. "Health Systems and the Right to Health: An Assessment of 194 Countries." *The Lancet* 372: 2047–85.

Bauhoff, S., D. Hotchkiss, and O. Smith. 2010. "The Impact of Medical Insurance for the Poor in Georgia: A Regression Discontinuity Approach." *Health Economics* 20: 1362–78.

Brinkerhoff, D. W. 2004. "Accountability and Health Systems: Toward Conceptual Clarity and Policy Relevance." *Health Policy and Planning* 19: 371–79.

Brinkerhoff, D. W., and T. R. Bossert. 2014. "Health Governance: Principal–Agent Linkages and Health System Strengthening." *Health Policy and Planning* 29 (6): 685–93.

Chevalier, F., P. Garel, and J. Levitan. 2009. *Hospitals in the 27 Member States of the European Union*. Paris: Dexia.

Devarajan, S., S. Khemani, and S. Shah. 2007. "The Politics of Partial Decentralization." World Bank.

Gauri, V., and D. Brinks. 2008. *Courting Social Justice: Judicial Enforcement of Social and Economic Rights in the Developing World*. Cambridge, UK: Cambridge University Press.

Iunes, R., L. Cubillos-Turriago, and M.-L. Escobar. 2012. "Universal Health Coverage and Litigation in Latin America." En Breve, World Bank,

Washington, DC. https://openknowledge.worldbank.org/handle/10986/13072 License: CC BY 3.0 IGO.

Leonard, K., P. Serneels, and M. Brock. 2013. "Intrinsic Motivation." In *The Labor Market for Health Workers in Africa: A New Look at the Crisis*, edited by A. Soucat, R. Scheffler, and T. A. Ghebreyesus, 255–284. Washington, DC: World Bank.

Paris, V., M. Devaux, and L. Wei. 2010. "Health System Institutional Characteristics: A Survey of 29 OECD Countries." Health Working Paper 50, Organisation for Economic Co-Operation and Development, Paris.

Peabody, J., M. M. Taguiwalo, D. A. Robalino, and J. Frenk. 2006. "Improving the Quality of Care in Developing Countries." In *Disease Control Priorities in Developing Countries*, edited by D. Jamison, J. G. Breman, A. R. Measham, G. Alleyene, M. Claeson, and D. B. Evans, 1293–308. Oxford: Oxford University Press.

Preker, A., and A. Harding, eds. 2003. *Innovations in Health Service Delivery: The Corporatization of Public Hospitals*. Washington, DC: World Bank.

Pritchett, Lant. 2002. "It Pays to Be Ignorant: A Simple Political Economy of Rigorous Program Evaluation." *Journal of Policy Reform* 5 (4): 251–69.

Ringold, D., A. Holla, M. Koziol, and S. Srinivasan. 2012. *Citizens and Service Delivery: Assessing the Use of Social Accountability Approaches in Human Development*. Washington, DC: World Bank.

Rockefeller Foundation, Save the Children, UNICEF, and World Health Organization. 2013. *Universal Health Coverage: A Commitment to Close the Gap*. London: Save the Children.

Rumbold, Benedict, Vidhya Alakeson, and Peter C. Smith. 2012. *Rationing Health Care: Is It Time to Set Out More Clearly What Is Funded by the NHS?* London: Nuffield Trust.

Saltman, R. B., A. Duran, and H. Dubois. 2011. *Governing Public Hospitals: Reform Strategies and the Movement towards Institutional Autonomy*. Copenhagen: European Observatory.

Wagstaff, Adam. 2010. "Social Health Insurance Reexamined." *Health Economics* 19 (5): 503–17.

WHO (World Health Organization). 2000. *World Health Report 2000*. Geneva: WHO.

———. 2007. *Everybody's Business: Strengthening Health Systems to Improve Health Outcomes*. Geneva: WHO.

———. 2014. "Making Fair Choices on the Path to UHC." http://apps.who.int/iris/bitstream/10665/112671/1/9789241507158_eng.pdf?ua=1.

World Bank. 2003. *World Development Report 2004: Making Services Work for Poor People*. Washington, DC: World Bank.

————. 2008. "Realizing Rights through Social Guarantees: An Analysis of New Approaches to Social Policy in Latin America and South Africa." Report 40047-GLB, Social Development Department, World Bank, Washington, DC.

————. 2014. "Opening the Black Box: Contextual Drivers of Social Accountability Effectiveness." World Bank, Washington, DC.

World Bank and WHO (World Health Organization). 2014. "Monitoring Progress towards Universal Health Coverage at Country and Global Levels: Framework, Measures and Targets." http://apps.who.int/iris /bitstream/10665/112824/1/WHO_HIS_HIA_14.1_eng.pdf?ua=1.

CHAPTER 7

Conclusions

Around the world, countries are implementing ambitious universal health coverage (UHC) programs. This study analyzed 26 UHC programs in 24 developing countries to understand in detail *how* these programs are implemented. The programs were selected on the basis that they followed a "bottom-up approach" toward UHC; they expanded coverage with a special focus on the poor, sharing the ultimate goal of ensuring that everyone has access to the health care they need without suffering financial hardship.

These programs are at once new, massive, and transformational: *new* because they have mostly been launched since the turn of the century; *massive* because they cover almost 2.5 billion people (and counting), or about one-third of the global population; and *transformational* in that they do not just expand coverage but fundamentally change the way that broader health systems work.

This concluding chapter briefly discusses the common policy elements observed across the 24 countries, the key policy choices that countries make in order to chart their own path toward UHC, the stepping stones they often use along that path, and the new risks that must be addressed.

Policy Convergence, Implementation Variations

The study aimed to find areas of policy convergence across the UHC programs. All of them are attempting to address both a financing gap by spending additional resources in a pro-poor way and a provision gap by seeking to change incentives in the service delivery domain. Countries are adopting two broad approaches to bottom-up UHC implementation. The first, referred to here as "supply-side programs," channels investments to expand the capacity of service provision through more funding for inputs (like human resources) and to promote reforms such as greater flexibility in staff recruitment, financial autonomy for public clinics, strong organizational protocols, and explicit performance indicators. The Universal Health Coverage Studies Series (UNICO) study covers eight such programs. They are "bottom up" because they focus on the services typically used by the poor—in six out of eight countries, the focus is on primary care.

The second broad approach is "demand-side programs" that attach resources to an identified population and to the services they use. These programs first identify and enroll their target population, prioritizing the poor and vulnerable and then they purchase health care services on their behalf usually via output-based pay. There are 18 such programs in the study.

These two approaches can complement each other on the road to UHC, although as explained below, the study found few countries implementing them at the same time.

The study analyzed the new tools and institutions reshaping health systems. By chapter, the analysis included the way systems cover people; expand and purchase health care benefits; manage money; improve health care provision; and hold actors at each level of the system accountable. Let us take a look at trends in each of these categories.

Covering People

The bottom-up approach is based on the recognition that different strategies are required to attend to the specific needs of each subpopulation. This requires overcoming the anonymity that typically characterized the relation of health systems with poor citizens. New citizen-identification systems being adopted in most countries, alongside new capacities for individual and geographic targeting, as well as better targeting registries identifying poor and vulnerable households, let governments differentially treat the poor and vulnerable, and target fiscal subsidies to them. These systems also let programs covering the nonpoor informal sector work better.

Expanding Benefits

The new UHC programs aim to improve and expand access to certain health care benefits by moving beyond coverage of the millennium development goal (MDG) interventions. They often make explicit the benefit package covered by the program. The more advanced countries among the 24 set down waiting times, draft specific clinical protocols, and establish a maximum financial risk to be borne by patients. To administer the package, many UHC programs also develop new systems of contracts and introduce new payment systems linking payments to successful delivery of benefits in the package.

Managing Money

The way money is managed for these programs changes the sources of funds and the way resources are pooled and allocated. In all countries, the expansion of coverage to the poor and vulnerable was noncontributory and fully tax financed. There is also a strong trend in that program financing is incremental, complementing rather than replacing traditional supply-side financing modalities. Further, the additional funds are not in most countries added to the historical budgets that fund payrolls and other inputs for public providers; instead, the new payments are linked to outputs (the services received by the population). This often leads to a new setup characterized by the coexistence of supply-side historical budgets for inputs and demand-side payments linked to outputs, and some countries have leveraged this arrangement to good effect.

Improving Health Care Provision

Many changes involving health care providers are being felt, which is good news because health care provision is a concern in many UNICO countries. One shift is that many UHC programs are attempting to inject greater flexibility not just into hiring health workers, but also into managing public clinics and hospitals, so as to make these facilities better able to respond to the new system of provider payments. This usually involves giving managers access to some "flexible" cash that can be rapidly allocated to operational needs or as incentives for staff and managers—or a bit of both. About half the 26 UHC programs are also expanding their capacity to provide more and better services by engaging with private providers. Effective coverage and quality are always a concern, to which most countries are responding by building or strengthening their systems of accreditation, setting the right conditions for the new output-based payments to work well.

Strengthening Accountability

The above measures aim to change the way stakeholders interact, strengthening accountability among policy makers, providers, and the population. Four instruments are being adopted—or reinforced—to enhance accountability: delegation (more arm's-length relationships together with more explicit identification of roles and responsibilities); financing (shift toward output-based financing); information and enforcement (greater data collection for UHC programs); and empowering citizens to achieve greater voice.

Policy Choices and Paths to UHC

Each country must beat its own path to UHC, to do so they must make some fundamental policy choices, and here we highlight five. *First* is whether to choose a bottom-up approach or not. While the study focused on countries that have opted for this approach, other countries may decide that "coverage" is not their primary health sector challenge (such as the countries of the former Soviet Union with overbuilt health systems), or that they are satisfied with the progress they have achieved expanding coverage through more traditional forms of organization (some highly equitable health systems such as those in Cuba, Malaysia, and Sri Lanka fall in this category). Some countries that have not yet chosen to expand coverage in earnest may decide that they do not have all the technical, political, and financial resources to follow the bottom-up path, and that if they did, they could put previous achievements at risk.

For countries choosing the bottom-up approach, once the poor have been covered a *second* area of policy choice is how to cover the nonpoor informal sector. In all countries coverage of the poor and vulnerable is noncontributory and covered by tax revenues, yet policy makers often hit a fork in the road when deciding how to cover the nonpoor informal sector. Some countries go along the contributory path, while others expand tax subsidies to everyone in the informal sector. Each path has pros and cons: the noncontributory path is faster but—for countries using a social health insurance (SHI) system for the formal sector—it creates a trade-off between equity and sustainability that may require profound tax and health reforms down the road. The contributory path is slower, as it requires front-loading reforms, but by avoiding the use of transitory steps, it creates a more stable and sustainable institutional setup.

Third, often closely tied to the non-/contributory choice, is how to pool resources for the various subpopulations. Some countries embed programs for the poor and vulnerable within their SHI agency, while others create autonomous programs for the poor and vulnerable and for the rest of the informal sector. While the use of a single pool has potential advantages for equity, in practice the single pool does not always produce more equitable results.

A *fourth* area relates to the path of expansion of the health care benefits financed by UHC programs. Most UNICO countries use UHC programs to strengthen services linked to the MDGs but aim to expand the benefits beyond the scope of MDG programs. Countries here face tough choices of what additions to prioritize. Consensus seems to have coalesced around the components of the initial package, but far less is apparent on the direction after that. Many countries have expanded benefits by including inpatient hospital benefits; others choose specialist outpatient benefits; and others emphasize expanding the list of eligible drugs or access to certain high-cost tertiary care services.

Fifth, countries also choose between supply- or demand-side UHC programs. In principle, they can do both as these programs can be complementary and do not reflect a choice of path—regardless of the path chosen, all countries need, for instance, a strong PHC pillar. In practice, however, few UNICO countries could implement significant reforms in both spheres simultaneously.

Stepping Stones

The methodology used by the study—comparing a large number of countries and looking in detail at the architecture and history of specific programs used by those countries—gives this book a special viewpoint. Not only does it have a cross-section of interventions that can be compared, but it also lets us understand some aspects of that cross-section by looking at the historical trajectory of individual programs. One key conclusion stems from this viewpoint: countries often make choices that would be imperfect for a final configuration of a health system providing universal health coverage, but that make sense if understood as temporary solutions.

Programs targeting the poor and vulnerable are sometimes criticized as being incompatible with UHC. Critics argue that universality requires covering all populations, including the informal sector, and that programs targeted to the poor are underfinanced and often result in low-quality services. Many countries use these programs as a starting point and then expand the program in different directions. The programs are useful stepping stones that give countries the opportunity to develop new skills in targeting, enrollment, output-based payments, and results-based budgeting.

Autonomous informal sector programs, operating separately from social health insurance, may also be transitory. They have advantages, including the capacity for rapid expansion, but they generate a trade-off between equity and sustainability, which, in the long run, may require additional reforms. One such path of reform—adoption of a fully tax-financed model—was followed by some UNICO countries (and by some high-income countries). Other countries may choose a contributory path.

Voluntary health insurance is often criticized for its inability to provide universal health coverage. This study's perspective suggests that it may serve a valuable purpose as a temporary solution providing some coverage and a smoother political transition than inaction in relation to the needs of the nonpoor informal sector population during the period when the focus of action of the government is on the poor and vulnerable.

Lastly, the coexistence of supply-side subsidies and demand-side payments may also be a transitory arrangement. While the introduction of demand-side payments improves incentives, it is unclear how well the different sources of funds are being combined at the local and the facility level.

So, some transitory steps are useful stepping stones, allowing countries to advance toward UHC, but more research is needed to identify which of them allow countries to retain flexibility in designing future steps, and which ones curtail it, creating path dependence. The experience of the UNICO countries suggests that starting narrow and then broadening (from targeting the poor to broader population coverage) is relatively easy to do; starting broad and later narrowing (from having a wide benefit package and then curtailing items) is much harder.

New Risks

New approaches entail new risks—in three areas. First, new programs are more complex and demand sophisticated technical and political capacities. Second, they involve explicit promises that generate expectations and create the risk of "broken promises" where actual outcomes fall short of expectations. Third, they may affect fiscal sustainability.

Increased Complexity

The UHC programs are not just about adding more resources to the system, but instead involve an attempt to introduce a new way of doing business which is more complex and requires new technical skills. The greater complexity is partly due to new activities that were not performed before, such as identifying and targeting subpopulations, enrolling in public programs, explicitly prioritizing certain health care services, or monitoring outputs by public providers. It is also in part due to new ways of implementing existing activities, such as operating with output-based payments, combining demand and supply finances, introducing financial audits, delivering services with patient-centered teamwork for chronic patients, or involving a third party for accrediting health care facilities.

The new programs also compel greater political skills, as they aim to change the way health systems are organized, generating winners and losers and thus requiring high-order political skills. These skills will be put to the test in, say, adopting explicit targeting; choosing the benefit-package expansion path from among those already supported by strong provider interest-groups; balancing short-term political gains secured through populist promises against long-term risks of sustainability; or bringing powerful new players (such as the pharmaceutical industry or associations of specialists in tertiary care) into day-to-day decision making on budget allocations.

Expectations versus Actual Outcomes and Broken Promises

The UHC programs make intensive use of new arrangements that require expectations to be set and outcomes (tied to those expectations) to be measured.

The study, unsurprisingly, found gaps between expectations and outcomes, notably that between the promised benefit package and the de facto benefits obtained by program beneficiaries. Significant implicit rationing of the promised benefit package occurs due to inadequate provider availability, geographic access issues, crowding at facilities offering these services, quantitative restrictions at health care providers, and long waiting periods. All this generates implicit rationing.

In terms of targeting, the transition is also slow and incomplete, generating a gap between theoretical and real-life arrangements. These challenges partly explain why the process of reaching significant proportions of the poor tends to be slower than envisaged. It also explains why many UHC programs continue to rely on mechanisms of self-selection, such as programs that allow contributory members the use of private providers but limit poor beneficiaries to the use of less attractive public providers.

Yet outcomes and expectations are rarely compared, even though large volumes of data are collected on multiple aspects of UHC programs. At their best, data can be pivotal in directing program course (as with performance indicators in Argentina and Brazil to determine intergovernmental fiscal transfers, or the growing use of technical and medical audits). But the wealth of data (sometimes due to the switch to output-based payments) is largely left unexploited, despite the data's potential value for managing cost or quality of provision, incidence of public expenditures on different subpopulations, or share of funds allocated to prioritized health benefits.

More generally, the lack of monitoring and reporting is also wide-spread: fewer than half the UHC programs include regular reporting on health outcomes and even fewer report on progress on financial protection and equity.

Fiscal Sustainability

Most UHC program expenditures are not excessive because they operate as discrete demand-side additions to existing supply-side public financing and, in some cases, are complemented by private out-of-pocket expenditure (OOPE) (by design).

The move toward making benefit packages more explicit potentially exposes countries to fiscal sustainability risks—for instance, from cost pressures, increased utilization rates, and adoption of expensive medicines and technology in the future—especially as accountability mechanisms mature in countries that lag behind. Some UNICO countries have mitigated fiscal sustainability risks by explicitly limiting or clearly circumscribing the benefits provided.

However, fiscal sustainability risks still loom large for countries that may have promised open-ended comprehensive entitlements that are not explicit, even if they are not, in effect, made universally available to all beneficiaries via implicit rationing that, typically, disproportionately affects the poor and vulnerable. In the short term, the fiscal risks in such countries may be low if this implicit rationing continues. However, in the longer term, benefits may need to be made more explicit.

Final Words ...

As noted at the start of this book, the journey toward UHC is a long one. Over the past decade or more, 24 countries have taken enormous strides toward achieving UHC through the launch of bottom-up programs aimed at the poor. Their progress over this time in the pursuit of a pro-poor health agenda has arguably been greater than during any previous decade. But the agenda remains incomplete, and some of our global lessons from the recent past can, we hope, when adapted to the results of a new generation of operational research, help countries chart an even more successful path toward UHC.

Universal Health Coverage Studies Series—Studies and Authors

No.	Title	Author(s)
1	The Mexican Social Protection System in Health	M.E. Bonilla-Chacin and Nelly Aguilera
2	Brazil's Primary Care Strategy	Bernard Couttolenc and Tania Dmytraczenko
3	Toward Synergy and Collaboration to Expand the Supply of and Strengthen Primary Health Care in Nigeria's Federal Context, with Special Reference to Ondo State	Chris Atim and Aarushi Bhatnagar
4	Consolidation and Transparency: Transforming Tunisia's Health Care for the Poor	Chokri Arfa and Heba Elgazzar
5	Improving Universal Primary Health Care by Kenya: A Case Study of the Health Sector Services Fund	Gandham N.V. Ramana
6	Jamaica's Effort in Improving Universal Access within Fiscal Constraints	Shiyan Chao
7	The Nuts & Bolts of Jamkesmas, Indonesia's Government-Financed Health Coverage Program	Pandu Harimurti, Eko Pambudi, Anna Pigazzini, and Ajay Tandon
8	The Long March to Universal Coverage: Lessons from China	Lilin Liang and John C. Langenbrunner
9	The Health Extension Program in Ethiopia	Netsanet W. Workie and Gandham N.V. Ramana
10	Peru's Comprehensive Health Insurance and New Challenges for UC	Pedro Francke
11	Argentina: Increasing Utilization of Health Care Services among the Uninsured Population: The Plan Nacer Program	Rafael Cortez and Daniela Romero
12	Expanding Health Coverage for Vulnerable Groups in India	Somil Nagpal

No.	Title	Author(s)
13	Costa Rica Case Study: Primary Health Care Achievements and Challenges within the Framework of the Social Health Insurance	Fernando Montenegro Torres
14	Colombia Case Study: The Subsidized Regime of Colombia's National Health Insurance System	Fernando Montenegro Torres, Fernando Acevedo, and Oscar Bernal
15	Georgia's Medical Insurance Program for the Poor	Owen Smith
16	Toward Universal Coverage in Health: The Case of the State Guaranteed Benefit Package of the Kyrgyz Republic	Antonio Giuffrida, Melitta Jakab, and Elina Dale
17	Turkey's Green Card Program for the Poor	Rekha Menon, Salih Mollahaliloglu, and Iryna Postolovska
18	Improving Access to Health Care Services through the Expansion of Coverage Program (PEC): The Case of Guatemala	Christine Lao Pena
19	Health Financing Reform in Thailand: Toward Universal Coverage under Fiscal Constraints	Piya Hanvoravongchai
20	Explicit Health Guarantees for Chileans: The Auge Benefits Package	Ricardo Bitran
21	The Philippines' Government Sponsored Health Coverage Program for Poor Households	Sarbani Chakraborty
22	Integrating the Poor into a Universal Health Program in Ghana (draft)	Karima Saleh
23	Integrating the Poor into Universal Health Coverage in Vietnam	Aparnaa Somanathan, Huong Lan Dao, and Tran Van Tien
24	The Impact of Universal Coverage Schemes in the Developing World: A Review of the Existing Evidence	Ursula Giedion, Eduardo Andrés Alfonso (who also updated the analysis), and Yadira Díaz
25	Comparing Comparisons: A Literature Review of Previous Attempts to learn from Comparative Studies (draft)	Ha Thi Hong Nguyen
26	The Antiretroviral Treatment Program in South Africa (draft)	Patrick Osewe and Hannah Kikaya

Source: http://www.worldbank.org/en/topic/health/publication/universal-health-coverage-study-series.
Note: Integral to the above UNICO studies is the questionnaire in appendix D.

UNICO Country Context

This annex summarizes key attributes of countries in the Universal Health Coverage Studies Series (UNICO), providing country context and comparisons with non-UNICO developing countries and with high-income countries. The UNICO study was of 24 countries: nine from the Latin America and the Caribbean (LAC) region; five each from the East Asia and Pacific (EAP) and Sub-Saharan Africa (SSA) regions; three from the Europe and Central Asia (ECA) region; and one country each from the South Asia (SAR) and Middle East and North Africa (MNA) regions (table B.1).

UNICO included countries that were some of the most populous in the world (China, India, and Indonesia) as well as three with populations of fewer than 5 million (Costa Rica, Georgia, and Jamaica). The total population in all 24 UNICO countries amounted to 4 billion, more than half the world's population in 2011. Less than half (44 percent) of the population was rural, compared with 53 percent in non-UNICO developing countries. With more than 80 percent of the population residing in rural areas, Ethiopia was the most rural. Argentina was the most urban, with less than 10 percent of its population living in rural areas. Table B.2 summarizes some key sociodemographic indicators across UNICO countries as of 2011, the year for which UNICO data were compiled.

The age distribution of the population is important in influencing the utilization of health care services: younger and older subgroups generally tend to have much higher rates. Georgia and Argentina were the only two UNICO countries with more than 10 percent of the population 65 years and older (table B.2). Lower-income UNICO countries generally had relatively lower proportion of the elderly population but a relatively larger share that was younger than 15: Ethiopia, Guatemala, Kenya, and Nigeria each had more than 40 percent of the population

TABLE B.1
Regional Distribution of UNICO Countries

Region	UNICO countries	All
EAP	China; Indonesia; Philippines; Thailand; Vietnam	5
ECA	Georgia; Kyrgyz Republic; Turkey	3
LAC	Argentina; Brazil; Chile; Colombia; Costa Rica; Guatemala; Jamaica; Mexico; Peru	9
MNA	Tunisia	1
SAR	India	1
SSA	Ethiopia; Ghana; Kenya; Nigeria; South Africa	5
All		24

aged 0–14 years. Three EAP UNICO countries—China, Thailand, and Vietnam—had the lowest overall age-dependency ratios (the combined share of the population younger than 15 or 65 years and older) across UNICO countries.

The average educational attainment in UNICO countries was 12.5 years, over one year more than in non-UNICO developing countries. With less than 10 years of schooling on average, Ethiopia and Nigeria had the lowest average educational attainment in the 24 UNICO countries; at 16.1 years, Argentina had the highest. Brazil, Chile, and Tunisia also had relatively higher educated populations, averaging more than 14 years of schooling.

Most UNICO countries have relatively democratic political systems. Chile and Costa Rica are the most democratic, followed by Turkey, Jamaica, Peru, India, and South Africa (figure B.1). The average "polity score" for UNICO countries was 5.8, more than double the corresponding average of 2.4 among non-UNICO developing countries (Marshall, Gurr, and Jaggers 2014).[1]

Macroeconomic Indicators

All UNICO countries had a gross domestic product (GDP) per capita of less than US$15,000 in 2011; among the 24 UNICO countries was one high-income country (Chile), 12 upper middle-income countries, 8 lower middle-income countries, and 3 low-income countries. Ethiopia was

TABLE B.2
Key Sociodemographic Indicators in UNICO Countries, 2011

Country	Population Millions	Rural (%)	Age 0–14 (%)	Age 15–64 (%)	Age 65+ (%)	Average years of schooling
Argentina	41	7.5	24.6	64.6	10.7	16.1
Brazil	200	15.4	25.0	67.9	7.1	14.2
Chile	17	10.9	21.7	68.8	9.4	14.7
China	1,300	49.5	18.0	73.5	8.5	11.7
Colombia	46	24.7	28.4	65.8	5.8	13.6
Costa Rica	4.7	35.4	24.4	68.9	6.7	13.7
Ethiopia	84	83.0	43.9	52.8	3.3	8.7
Georgia	4.5	47.1	17.4	68.4	14.2	13.2
Ghana	25	48.1	38.8	57.7	3.5	11.4
Guatemala	15	50.2	41.2	54.4	4.5	10.7
India	1,220	68.7	29.8	65.1	5.1	10.7
Indonesia	240	49.3	29.6	65.3	5.1	12.9
Jamaica	2.7	47.9	28.4	63.7	7.9	13.1
Kenya	42	76.0	42.5	54.9	2.6	11.1
Kyrgyz Republic	5.5	64.6	30.1	65.6	4.3	12.6
Mexico	120	21.9	29.5	64.3	6.1	13.7
Nigeria	160	50.4	44.1	53.1	2.7	9.0
Peru	29	22.8	29.6	64.3	6.1	13.2
Philippines	95	51.1	34.9	61.3	3.8	11.7
South Africa	51	38.0	29.6	65.1	5.3	13.1
Thailand	67	65.9	18.9	72.0	9.1	12.3
Tunisia	11	33.7	23.3	69.7	7.0	14.5
Turkey	73	28.6	26.4	66.5	7.2	12.9
Vietnam	88	69.0	23.1	70.3	6.5	11.9
UNICO countries	4,000 (total)	44.2	29.3	64.3	6.4	12.5
Non-UNICO developing countries	1,700 (total)	52.6	34.0	60.6	5.4	11.1
High-income countries	1,260 (total)	25.0	18.5	68.8	12.7	12.7

Source: WDI.

FIGURE B.1
Democratization, UNICO Countries, 2011

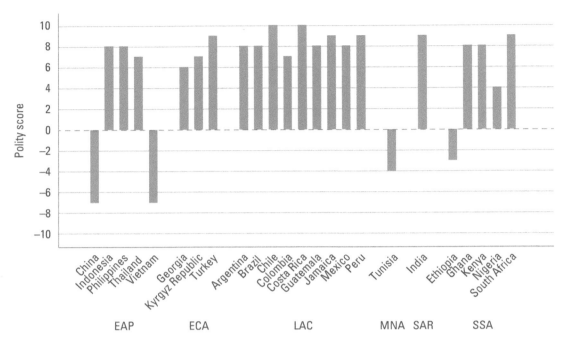

Source: Polity IV Project.
Note: Autocracies –10 to –6; anocracies –5 to 5; democracies 6 to 10.

the poorest country, with a GDP per capita of only US$335; Chile was the richest, with a GDP per capita of US$14,513 (figure B.2). UNICO countries represent a relatively richer subset of developing countries: the median GDP per capita across them was about US$4,771 in 2011; by way of contrast, the median GDP per capita among non-UNICO developing countries was about US$3,022.[2]

There were significant variations in the extent of nationally defined poverty rates across UNICO countries. A third or more of the population was classified by governments as poor in Guatemala, Kenya, the Kyrgyz Republic, Mexico, and Nigeria; and about a quarter to a third of the population in Colombia, Ethiopia, Ghana, Peru, and the Philippines (table B.3). Less than 15 percent of the population was classified as poor in Chile, China, Georgia, Indonesia, and Thailand. The proportion of the nationally defined population classified as poor was not strongly correlated with GDP per capita.

On internationally comparable absolute poverty rates, in Ethiopia, India, and Kenya more than 60 percent of the population—in Nigeria more than 80 percent—lived on less than $2 a day circa 2011 (Figure B.3).

FIGURE B.2
Income and Income Classification of UNICO Countries, 2011

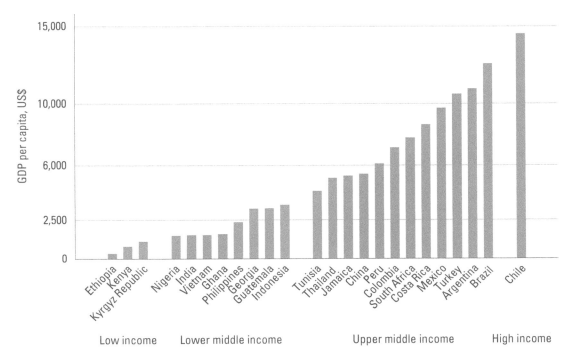

Source: WDI.

Nigeria and Kenya were two countries that also had the largest shares (>40 percent) of their populations living on less than $1 a day, the Millennium Development Goal (MDG) benchmark for absolute poverty. More than a third of the population lived on less than $1 a day in Ethiopia, India, and Ghana. In almost all upper middle-income UNICO countries (China and South Africa being exceptions) less than 20 percent of the population lived on less than $2 a day. The median $1-a-day and $2-a-day poverty rates among UNICO countries were 10 percent and 24 percent, respectively (lower than the median numbers for non-UNICO countries, which were 12 percent and 27 percent, respectively).

South Africa was the most unequal country on income distribution: the bottom 40 percent of its population accounted for only 19 percent of consumption. Most LAC countries were also relatively unequal, giving the region the highest regional Gini index average (figure B.4). The least unequal countries were, in ascending order, the Kyrgyz Republic, Ethiopia, and India. In the Kyrgyz Republic, the bottom 40 percent of the population accounted for 30 percent of all consumption.

TABLE B.3
Nationally Defined Poverty Rates in UNICO Countries, circa 2011

<15% poor	≥15% to <25% poor	≥25% to <33% poor	≥33% poor
China; Indonesia; Thailand; Chile; Georgia	Tunisia; Brazil; Vietnam; Jamaica; Turkey; Costa Rica; India; South Africa	Philippines; Peru; Ghana; Ethiopia; Colombia	Kyrgyz Republic; Kenya; Nigeria; Mexico; Guatemala

FIGURE B.3
Absolute Poverty Rates in UNICO Countries, circa 2011

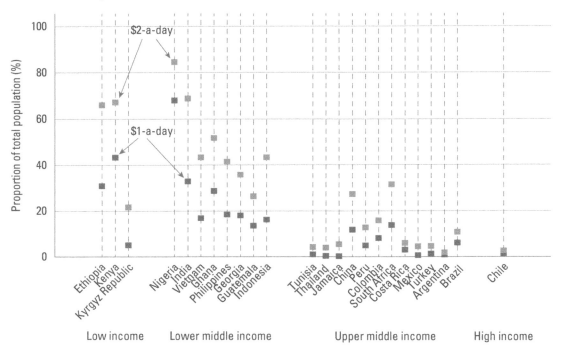

Source: WDI.

UNICO countries generally grew faster than non-UNICO countries over the past decade or so. Economic growth averaged 4.3 percent per year over 2000–12 among UNICO countries; the non-UNICO developing country rate was 3.8 percent (figure B.5). However, economic growth was relatively more volatile among UNICO countries, notably during the 2008–09 global financial crisis.

Economic growth can be an important enabling factor for financing expansion in universal health coverage (UHC), especially if other

FIGURE B.4
Distribution of Gini Index across UNICO Countries, 2011

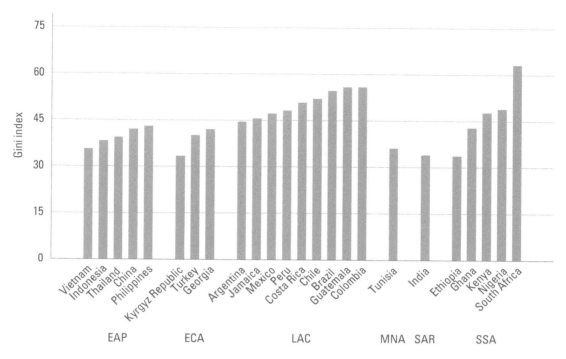

Source: WDI.

macroeconomic indicators such as deficit and debt are not too high and health is accorded priority over other sectors by the government. Over the reference period 2000–12, more than two-thirds of UNICO countries had average deficits of less than 3 percent of GDP and average debt of less than 60 percent of GDP (figure B.6).[3] Seven of the 24 UNICO countries had deficits greater than 3 percent of GDP and debt levels higher than 60 percent of GDP: Jamaica, the Kyrgyz Republic, Ethiopia, India, Argentina, Brazil, and Ghana.

Key Population Health Outcomes

In 2011 there was wide variation in life expectancy rates among the UNICO countries: Costa Rica (80 years) and Chile (79) had the highest life expectancies, almost the same as the median for high-income countries (80); Nigeria and South Africa had the lowest (below 60). UNICO countries in 2011 had a median life expectancy of over 73 years, five years higher than non-UNICO developing countries (table B.4). Life

FIGURE B.5
Median GDP Growth in UNICO and Non-UNICO Developing Countries, 2000–12

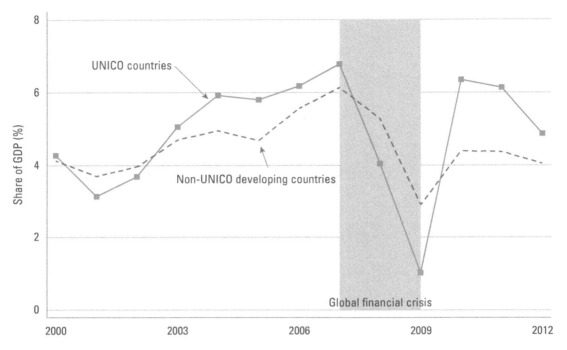

Source: WDI.

expectancy among UNICO countries was higher than non-UNICO countries even in 2000, before most UNICO countries had begun their UHC programs (figure B.7).

Around 2011 UNICO countries collectively had a median under-five mortality rate of 34 per 1,000 live births, better than the corresponding median among non-UNICO developing countries of 52 per 1,000 live births. As with life expectancy, Chile and Costa Rica had the best rates (and Nigeria the worst). Only about half the UNICO countries were on track for reducing under-five mortality by two-thirds over the 25-year MDG reference period (1990–2015). The median pace of decline in under-five mortality in UNICO countries over 2000–12 was 3.7 percent per year, higher than that among non-UNICO developing countries (3.2 percent). Some UNICO countries with relatively slow declines already had low baseline rates, such as Costa Rica and Chile. There was no systematic pattern in rates relative to income across UNICO countries: some positive outliers were Ethiopia and Vietnam; relatively large negative outliers were Nigeria and South Africa (figure B.8).

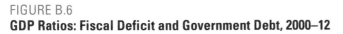

FIGURE B.6
GDP Ratios: Fiscal Deficit and Government Debt, 2000–12

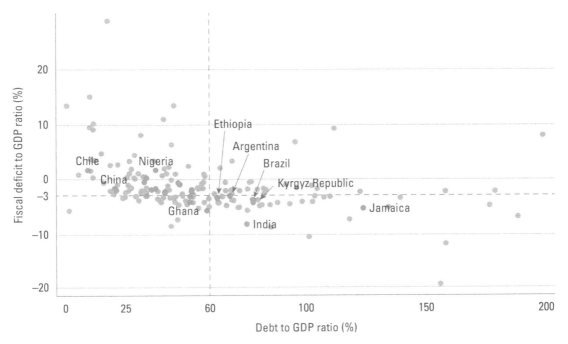

Source: IMF.
Note: UNICO countries highlighted.

As with under-five mortality, the maternal mortality ratio (MMR) was better in UNICO countries on average than among non-UNICO developing countries: 80 versus 137 maternal deaths per 100,000 live births, respectively. In order, Turkey, Chile, and Thailand were UNICO countries with the best MMRs, all under 30. Kenya, Ethiopia, and Nigeria had some of the worst MMRs, all exceeding 400. Unlike the case for under-five mortality, however, the average annual rate of decline in the MMR was about the same in UNICO countries as non-UNICO countries (table B.4). Two-thirds of UNICO countries had MMRs that were worse than expected for their income, notably Nigeria, Ghana, Indonesia, South Africa, and Brazil (figure B.8). Vietnam and the Kyrgyz Republic were two notable positive outliers.

Causes of the overall disease burden varied by income and region. Noncommunicable diseases were predominant causes of morbidity and mortality, accounting for more than 75 percent of all disability-adjusted life years (DALYs) lost in Georgia, Argentina, Chile, China, Costa Rica, and Turkey. Communicable diseases dominated the disease burden in SSA countries, as in Ethiopia, Ghana, Kenya, Nigeria, and

TABLE B.4
Key Population Health Indicators

Country	Life expectancy 2011	Under-five mortality rate		Maternal mortality ratio	
		2011	% rate of change (2000–12)	2011	% rate of change (2000–12)
Argentina	76	15	−2.9	74	1.1
Brazil	73	15	−6.7	68	−1.8
Chile	79	9	−1.5	23	−2.0
China	75	15	−7.8	35	−5.2
Colombia	74	18	−2.9	84	−3.6
Costa Rica	80	10	−2.3	35	−1.5
Ethiopia	62	72	−6.1	473	−6.4
Georgia	74	21	−4.4	42	−3.0
Ghana	61	74	−3.0	400	−3.1
Guatemala	71	33	−3.7	140	−1.1
India	66	59	−4.0	210	−5.0
Indonesia	70	32	−4.3	203	−3.7
Jamaica	73	17	−2.7	81	−0.7
Kenya	60	76	−3.4	440	−2.5
Kyrgyz Republic	70	28	−5.1	78	−2.2
Mexico	77	17	−3.7	48	−2.6
Nigeria	52	128	−3.4	593	−4.1
Peru	74	19	−6.3	96	−4.4
Philippines	68	31	−2.5	120	0.0
South Africa	55	47	−4.0	140	−0.6
Thailand	74	14	−4.4	27	−3.3
Tunisia	75	17	−5.0	47	−2.7
Turkey	75	15	−7.7	21	−3.8
Vietnam	76	23	−2.6	50	−4.1
UNICO countries	73	34	−3.8	80	−2.9
Non-UNICO developing countries	68	52	−3.7	137	−3.0
High-income countries	80	5	−3.2	10	−2.3

Source: WDI.

FIGURE B.7

Median Life Expectancy at Birth in UNICO and Non-UNICO Countries, 2000–12

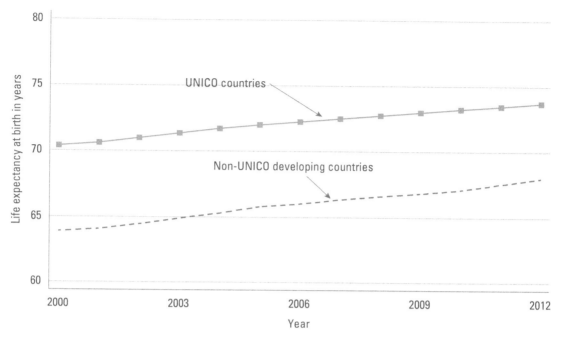

Source: WDI.

South Africa (table B.5). Ischemic heart disease was the biggest cause of the disease burden in eight UNICO countries; lower respiratory infections were the biggest cause in five; HIV/AIDS dominated in four countries; stroke was predominant in three. Interpersonal violence was the largest cause of DALYs in Colombia, malaria in Ghana, diabetes in Mexico, and preterm birth complications in India.

Health Financing

Despite being richer on average than other developing countries, UNICO countries spent a lower share of their GDP on health: total health expenditure (THE) as a share of GDP was 6.1 percent among UNICO countries versus 6.4 percent among non-UNICO developing countries (table B.6). Costa Rica, Georgia, Brazil, and South Africa had THE shares of GDP in excess of 8 percent; at less than 3 percent of GDP, Indonesia had the lowest share. Colombia and Thailand had the largest public share (exceeding 75 percent) of THE in the 24 countries; at 18.1 percent, Georgia had the lowest. The out-of-pocket (OOP) share of THE averaged 35.0 percent

FIGURE B.8
Under-Five Mortality Rate and Maternal Mortality Ratio Relative to Income, 2011

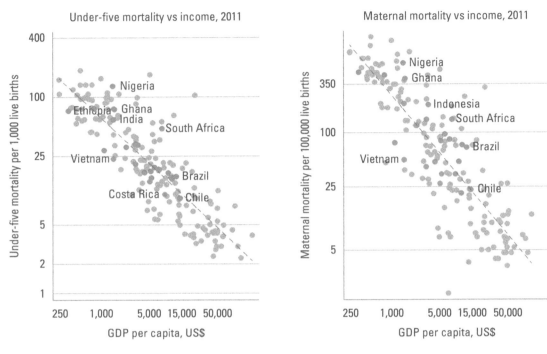

Source: WDI.
Note: UNICO countries highlighted; y-axis and x-axis log scale.

in UNICO countries (slightly lower than 38.2 percent among non-UNICO countries): the OOP share was highest, exceeding 60 percent, in Georgia and Nigeria (table B.6). Total and public health expenditures as a share of GDP grew at roughly the same pace among both UNICO and non-UNICO developing countries (figure B.9). The Philippines had the highest elasticity of THE to GDP over 1995–2012, Colombia the lowest. UNICO countries had a higher average share for health in the government budget (12.6 percent) than non-UNICO developing countries (10.7 percent).

Health Inputs and Coverage

Broad measures of health system inputs such as numbers of human resources for health (doctors, nurses, and midwives) and hospital beds per 1,000 population were, around 2011, generally higher in richer UNICO countries. Notable exceptions were the two ex-Soviet countries

TABLE B.5
Overall Disease Burden in UNICO Countries, 2010

Country	Share of burden of disease (%)			Top three causes of burden of disease		
	Noncom-municable	Commu-nicable	Injuries	#1	#2	#3
Argentina	76	13	11	Ischemic heart disease	Stroke	Major depressive disorder
Brazil	69	17	15	Ischemic heart disease	Interpersonal violence	Low back pain
Chile	79	9	13	Ischemic heart disease	Low back pain	Stroke
China	77	10	13	Stroke	Ischemic heart disease	COPD
Colombia	61	21	18	Interpersonal violence	Ischemic heart disease	Major depressive disorder
Costa Rica	77	12	12	Ischemic heart disease	Major depressive disorder	Low back pain
Ethiopia	28	63	9	Lower respiratory infections	Diarrheal diseases	Malaria
Georgia	81	11	8	Ischemic heart disease	Stroke	COPD
Ghana	34	60	6	Malaria	HIV/AIDS	Lower respiratory infections
Guatemala	46	37	17	Lower respiratory infections	Interpersonal violence	Diarrheal diseases
India	45	43	12	Preterm birth complications	Diarrheal diseases	Lower respiratory infections
Indonesia	58	33	9	Stroke	Tuberculosis	Road injury
Jamaica	64	23	13	HIV/AIDS	Diabetes	Stroke
Kenya	24	69	7	HIV/AIDS	Lower respiratory infections	Malaria
Kyrgyz Republic	58	29	13	Ischemic heart disease	Lower respiratory infections	Stroke
Mexico	71	15	13	Diabetes	Ischemic heart disease	Chronic kidney disease

table continues next page

TABLE B.5 *(Continued)*

Country	Share of burden of disease (%)			Top three causes of burden of disease		
	Noncom-municable	Commu-nicable	Injuries	#1	#2	#3
Nigeria	20	71	9	Lower respiratory infections	HIV/AIDS	Lower respiratory infections
Peru	62	28	10	Lower respiratory infections	Major depressive disorder	Ischemic heart disease
Philippines	58	33	9	Lower respiratory infections	Ischemic heart disease	Tuberculosis
South Africa	31	61	9	HIV/AIDS	Diarrheal diseases	Interpersonal violence
Thailand	66	19	14	HIV/AIDS	Ischemic heart disease	Road injury
Tunisia	72	16	12	Ischemic heart disease	Road injury	Major depressive disorder
Turkey	76	16	8	Ischemic heart disease	Stroke	Major depressive disorder
Vietnam	66	21	13	Stroke	Road injury	Low back pain

Source: Institute of Health Metrics and Evaluation Database.

among the UNICO countries, Georgia and the Kyrgyz Republic: both had the highest proportions of human resources for health and hospital beds per capita among all 24 countries (figure B.10). Ethiopia was a negative outlier with only 0.3 human resources for health per 1,000 population (far lower than the norm recommended by the World Health Organization [WHO] of 2.3) and 0.9 hospital beds per capita (also far below WHO's recommended 2.5). Most other UNICO countries were clustered around WHO norms for human resources and hospital beds, although India and Indonesia had very few hospital beds per capita.[4]

Ensuring that everyone has access to health care when needed, without experiencing financial hardship as a result—UHC—is typically conceptualized as having three key dimensions: *population coverage* (or "breadth" of coverage); *service coverage* (or "depth" of coverage); and *cost coverage* (or "height" of coverage). The UHC cube is one way of conceptualizing how far a country is from this three-dimensional ideal of everyone covered by all possible services without having to pay OOP (figure B.11) (WHO 2010).

TABLE B.6
Key Health Financing Indicators in UNICO Countries, 2011
Percent

Country	Total health expenditure share of GDP	Public share of total health expenditure	OOP share of total health expenditure
Argentina	7.9	66.5	21.0
Brazil	8.9	45.7	31.3
Chile	7.1	48.4	33.0
China	5.1	55.9	34.8
Colombia	6.5	75.2	15.9
Costa Rica	10.2	74.7	23.0
Ethiopia	4.1	50.0	39.9
Georgia	9.4	18.1	64.9
Ghana	5.3	55.9	29.8
Guatemala	6.7	35.4	53.3
India	3.9	30.5	59.9
Indonesia	2.9	37.9	47.4
Jamaica	5.2	53.6	32.9
Kenya	4.4	39.4	46.5
Kyrgyz Republic	6.2	59.9	34.5
Mexico	6.0	50.3	45.5
Nigeria	5.7	34.0	63.1
Peru	4.7	56.9	37.5
Philippines	4.4	36.9	52.7
South Africa	8.7	47.7	7.2
Thailand	4.1	77.7	12.4
Tunisia	7.0	59.4	35.2
Turkey	6.1	72.7	17.6
Vietnam	6.8	45.2	45.6
UNICO countries	6.1	50.2	35.0
Non-UNICO developing countries	6.0	53.6	38.2
High-income countries	7.2	72.5	18.8

Source: WDI.

FIGURE B.9
Total and Public Health Expenditure Share of GDP, 2000–12

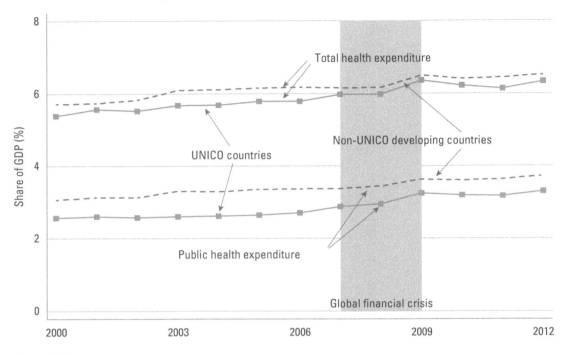

Source: WDI.

The three dimensions of UHC are neither independent nor mutually exclusive: ensuring depth of coverage has implications for the breadth and height of UHC as well. Universal availability of the benefit package for all—not just those who are well-off and live in urban areas—is a key aspect of ensuring that UHC is not a hypothetical aspiration but a realized policy designed to enhance health and improve financial protection. And high OOP payments—low height of UHC—is often a result of poor depth of coverage if patients have to pay OOP for drugs or seek care elsewhere in private facilities that are outside the network of UHC-eligible facilities.

Some UNICO countries such as Chile, China, Costa Rica, and Thailand already claim to provide universal or near-universal coverage for their citizens; others such as Indonesia and Vietnam cover half or more of their populations, with plans for expansion to reach universal coverage over the next five to six years. Population coverage is lower in some lower-income countries such as Ethiopia and Kenya, but even they have made progress in removing financial barriers for certain

FIGURE B.10

Human Resources for Health and Hospital Beds per 1,000 Population, circa 2011

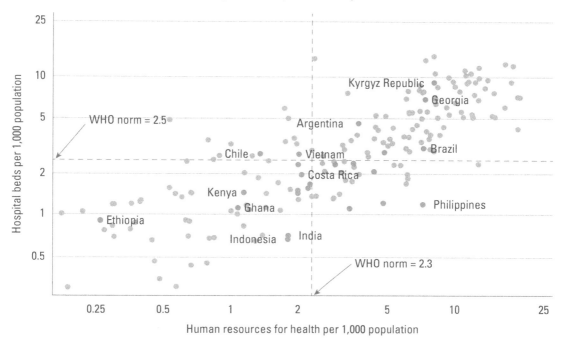

Source: WDI.
Note: Y-axis and x-axis log scale.

FIGURE B.11

The Three Dimensions of the UHC Cube

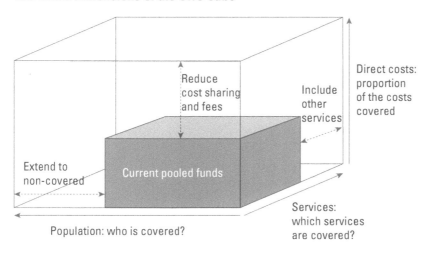

subgroups such as the poor, and for services related to maternal and child health.

The number of people covered is, of course, only one dimension. The 2014 joint WHO-World Bank framework for monitoring progress toward UHC recommends two sets of targets for assessing progress to UHC: at least 80 percent coverage of essential health services, regardless of level of wealth, place of residence, or gender; and 100 percent protection from both catastrophic and impoverishing health payments for the population as a whole, including for specified equity strata of the population (WHO and World Bank 2014).

For assessing the coverage of essential health services, the framework suggests the following 11 indicators: satisfaction of family planning needs; at least four antenatal care visits for pregnant women; measles vaccination in children; improved water source; adequate sanitation; nonuse of tobacco; skilled birth attendance during delivery; antiretroviral therapy; TB case detection and treatment success (combined into one indicator); hypertension treatment; and diabetes treatment. To measure the height of coverage, it suggests two indicators: proportion of households not incurring catastrophic payments; and the fraction of households that is neither impoverished by OOP payments nor pushed further into poverty by them. Cross-country comparable data are not yet available for all of these indicators and, in some cases, are available only for variations of recommended indicators (such as data on the proportion of pregnant women who had at least one antenatal care visit is available rather than on whether they had at least four antenatal care visits).[5]

Seven of the 11 essential health coverage indicators are in table B.7. About two-thirds of all UNICO countries had average coverage across all seven indicators greater than 80 percent. Coverage was particularly high in Costa Rica and Thailand, with average coverage in excess of 90 percent; at the low end were Ethiopia, Ghana, India, Kenya, and Nigeria, averaging below 70 percent. For most indicators, coverage rates were higher among UNICO countries than among non-UNICO developing countries.

TABLE B.7
Seven Essential Health Services Coverage Indicators, circa 2011
Percent

Country	Contra-ceptive prevalence rate	At least one an-tenatal care	Measles vaccina-tion rate	Access to improved water	Access to improved sanita-tion	Skilled birth atten-dance	TB detec-tion and treatment success rate
Argentina	78	91	94	99	97	97	47
Brazil	81	97	99	98	81	97	62
Chile	58	95	90	99	99	100	62
China	88	94	99	92	65	100	84
Colombia	79	97	94	91	80	99	58
Costa Rica	82	99	90	97	94	99	77
Ethiopia	29	34	66	52	24	10	61
Georgia	53	96	93	99	93	100	63
Ghana	34	90	88	87	14	68	68
Guatemala	54	93	93	94	80	52	29
India	55	75	74	93	36	52	53
Indonesia	62	93	80	85	59	83	63
Jamaica	72	99	93	93	80	98	27
Kenya	46	92	93	62	30	44	70
Kyrgyz Republic	36	97	98	88	92	99	61
Mexico	73	96	99	95	85	96	63
Nigeria	18	53	42	64	28	49	38
Peru	76	95	94	87	73	87	74
Philippines	49	91	85	92	74	72	68
South Africa	60	92	79	95	74	91	55
Thailand	80	99	98	96	93	100	68
Tunisia	63	96	96	97	90	99	82
Turkey	73	92	98	100	91	95	78
Vietnam	78	88	96	95	75	93	68
UNICO countries	62	89	89	89	71	83	53
Non-UNICO developing countries	43	86	86	82	61	77	62
High-income countries	69	100	95	100	100	100	62

Source: WDI.

Notes

1. The Polity Project estimates a polity score on a 21-point scale ranging from −10 (hereditary monarchy) to +10 (consolidated democracy) depending on the extent of democratization across countries. The 21-point score can be converted into three suggested regime categories: "autocracies" (−10 to −6), "anocracies" (−5 to +5), and "democracies" (+6 to +10).
2. The median GDP per capita in 1995 among UNICO countries was US$1,845, almost double that of non-UNICO developing countries.
3. The deficit and debt threshold benchmarks of 3 percent and 60 percent of GDP, respectively, are the macroeconomic Maastricht criteria for the European Union.
4. These low numbers may be an artifact of poor data quality, as information on private beds is often not readily available.
5. Systematic, comparable, and robust cross-country data on financial protection, particularly, are unavailable.

References

Marshall, M. G., T. R. Gurr, and K. Jaggers. 2014. "Polity IV Project: Political Regime Characteristics and Transitions 1800–2013." http://www .systemicpeace.org/polity/polity4.htm.

WHO (World Health Organization). 2010. *World Health Report 2010. Health Systems Financing: The Path to Universal Coverage.* Geneva: WHO.

WHO and World Bank. 2014. *Monitoring Progress towards Universal Health Coverage at Country and Global Levels.* Geneva: WHO.

The Impact of Universal Health Coverage Programs on Access, Financial Protection, and Health Status—A Literature Review

Introduction

Universal health coverage (UHC) is a key goal in many countries. This appendix reviews the literature on the impact of UHC programs on access, financial protection, and health status, synthesizing key findings and identifying gaps in knowledge for further research.

Impact of UHC Programs in a Nutshell

The impact evaluation literature finds that UHC programs *can* improve access, financial protection, and health status, but not all of them do. Some of the programs have the desired impact on access or financial protection, but not on health outcomes. Within the studies that find an impact, most find an increase in the utilization of some services but not others, improvement in some aspect of financial protection but not others, or improvement in only some of the health outcomes analyzed. There is also variation about who benefits: many of the programs have an impact on one subpopulation (often the poor) but not on others.

What this literature does not tell us is *why* some programs have an impact and others do not. This limits the operational usefulness of this type of study as policy makers cannot learn from them *how* to design their programs. This limitation is due to two main factors. First, the programs operate in different contexts and the impact evaluation studies do not allow an understanding of what works in what context; the individual studies try to ascertain if "program X in context Y works" and are not designed to learn how program design needs to adapt to different contexts.

Second, even though the review focuses only on demand-side programs, each program involves numerous policies, and even though these policies have some characteristics in common across countries, the application of each policy varies by country in, for example: *How do programs cover people* (are they targeting just the poor and vulnerable or also covering the nonpoor informal sector?). *How do they expand benefits* (do they include inpatient care or only outpatient care? Do they contract providers using fee for service or other payment systems?). *How is the supply side organized and improved* (are there integrated networks, can private providers participate, do public providers have some autonomy?).

To respond to these and similar questions, a new generation of operational research needs to be developed; the new studies need a granular understanding of how policies are designed and what objective policy makers are trying to achieve when they choose one option over another. While this book does not attempt to measure the impact of the policies reviewed, it hopes to contribute to the development of a new operational research agenda by providing some of this needed granularity.

Methods

This appendix builds on previous literature reviews with related objectives (Giedion, Alfonso, and Diaz 2013; Giedion and Diaz 2008, 2011). For this synthesis, we updated the search and adjusted the eligibility criteria to include studies that examined the impact of UHC programs whose core component is a demand-side intervention aimed to reduce or eliminate payments at the point of service, including UHC programs labeled insurance, other programs that use prepayment and/or pooling to pay for health care instead of using direct payments, and voucher initiatives.[1] To identify studies, we also put together a list of UHC programs whose evaluations would be eligible for the review using initiatives frequently referred to as being part of the countries' UHC strategies.[2]

The studies typically use as a comparison group the people not directly affected by the UHC program, sometimes due to eligibility criteria, phased rollout of the program, differences in geographic placement, and similar arrangements to re-create a counterfactual.

To be included, a study must examine the impact of the UHC program on three outcomes: access to health care, financial protection, and health status. In this synthesis we focused on experimental and nonexperimental studies with an identification strategy using the methods discussed by

Gertler, Martinez, and Celhay (2011).[3] However, we did not include studies that used only matching methods, because the assumption that there are no unobserved factors affecting both participation and outcomes is unlikely to hold for most UHC programs. We only included instrumental variables (IV) studies in case of randomized design[4] or if IV is used in the context of a regression discontinuity approach.

We used automatic search in several databases[5] as well as hand search in a number of web pages[6] using two approaches: first, general terms for the intervention,[7] outcomes,[8] and methods[9] (this produced 6,579 records); and second, specific searches for the countries/UHC programs in our list of initiatives whose evaluations should be included in the review (which produced 281 additional records—see endnote 2). We also used one-way snowballing (cross-referencing from included studies, but not citation tracking) and in previous rounds of this review we also contacted key experts to ask for unpublished and ongoing studies that we may have missed. We included studies published and unpublished (book chapters, working papers) covering 2000–13. The results of the search and selection of studies are summarized in figure C.1.

FIGURE C.1
Selecting the Studies for Review

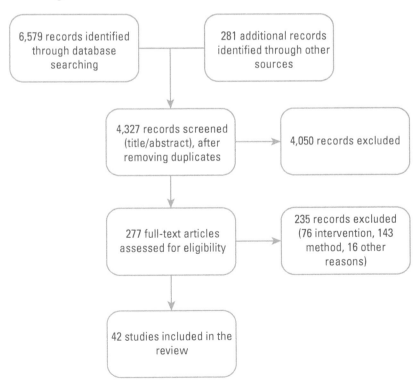

We screened 4,327 titles/abstracts, and after excluding 4,050 records (which did not include all the requisites described above), further assessed for eligibility 277 studies based on full-text inspection, and finally included in the review 42 studies that met all the inclusion criteria (in bold in the *References*). The studies cover 23 programs in 15 countries from most regions of the developing world. Given the diversity of interventions, outcome measures, units of measurement, methods, and parameters used in the literature, we chose to do a narrative review instead of a formal meta analysis.

The UHC Programs Evaluated

The UHC programs grouped above share some key traits, but differ in many others (see table C.1 for a complete list), including implementation details. The structure, prioritization of subpopulations, and contents of the benefit packages vary considerably. In addition, while all programs reviewed include a demand-side intervention, some of the programs also have strong supply-side components while others rely exclusively on demand-side interventions. The role of the private sector and the public network of providers also change considerably by program.

Among the UHC programs evaluated there are programs such as the Vietnam Health Insurance (VHI) that resemble a social health insurance (SHI) program. These are typically mandatory for formal sector employees and normally require explicit enrollment and payment of a contribution, which entitle beneficiaries to free access to health care, or at least user fees that are usually lower than they would have to pay elsewhere.

Another group comprises programs that are autonomous from SHI programs and targeted at the poor, the informal sector, or those otherwise uncovered. Examples include Colombia's Subsidized Regime, the Askeskin program in Indonesia, Mexico's Seguro Popular, and social security health insurance for Nicaragua's informal sector.

A number of community-based health insurance (CBHI) programs were evaluated. These programs are typically run at municipality, village, or small town level, and although they usually follow the same model, implementation details may vary. Participation is voluntary, membership is usually required and defined at the household level, and enrollees have to pay an insurance premium, although it is sometimes highly subsidized (either by government contributions or external donor funding). Examples of these programs are the CBHI program evaluated in Burkina Faso and China's New Cooperative Medical Scheme (NCMS), which also share some features such as voluntary participation, household enrollment, administration at the county level, and sometimes the payment of small insurance premiums that complement the funding of the program, consisting mainly of subsidies from the central and local governments.

A number of programs target a relatively narrow set of services, focusing on a few prioritized conditions such as maternal and newborn health. Examples of this include the Bangladesh voucher program and Plan Nacer in Argentina.

Does the Evidence Show Beneficial Impacts of UHC Programs?

Access—UHC Programs Can Improve Access, but Not All of Them Do, and It's Hard to Draw Lessons on Guidance for Implementation Elsewhere

Most studies use health care utilization as the primary outcome, including measures of general use of outpatient care, inpatient care, and utilization indicators of services for specific health conditions, such as maternity and newborn (prenatal care, institutional delivery, healthy-child checkups, etc.). The outcome measures differ in the units of measurement, including number of medical encounters, use of health care in the past year, probability of seeking care in case of need, and probability of using health care, among others. Table C.1 summarizes the key findings of the studies included in the review.

Several studies report mostly favorable impacts of the UHC programs on access. For example, Sparrow, Suryahadi, and Widyanti (2013) report positive impact of Askeskin in Indonesia on outpatient utilization. Nguyen et al. (2012) find that a maternal health voucher program in Bangladesh increases institutional delivery and delivery with qualified providers. Wagstaff and Pradhan (2005) find that VHI increases the use of primary care facilities for children and hospital services for children and adults. Gruber, Hendren, and Townsend (2012) report an increase in health care utilization brought about by Thailand's Universal Health Care Coverage Program (initially known as the 30-Baht program). Miller, Pinto, and Vera-Hernández (2009) conclude that the Subsidized Regime in Colombia has increased the use of health care, particularly for preventive services. Gertler, Martinez, and Celhay (2011) report that Plan Nacer in Argentina improves early detection of pregnant women, increases the number of prenatal care visits, and induces healthy-child checkups according to guidelines. Kraft et al. (2009) find that higher insurance coverage in the Philippines reduces the delays in seeking health care for children in need.

These and other studies report some form of improvement in access to health care due to the UHC programs. However, it would be wrong to conclude that any UHC program including a demand-side component to reduce the payments at the point of service would have such an effect, for several reasons.

First, several studies found no impact: Wagstaff (2010), for example, concludes there is no evidence that Vietnam's health care fund for the poor had any impact on utilization of health care, out- or inpatient. Nguyen (2012a), examining the impact of health insurance alternatives for children in Vietnam on annual outpatient contacts, reports no effects of the programs. King et al. (2009) find that after 10 months of implementation, Seguro Popular in Mexico did not have an impact on health care utilization. Robyn et al. (2012) for Burkina Faso analyzed health-seeking behavior for individuals reporting a health problem in the 30 days preceding the interview and they find no strong evidence of impact in a CBHI program.

There is even an example where the program may have *negatively* affected utilization: Wagstaff and Yu (2007) examine the impact of the World Bank's Health VIII project in Gansu province, China, a program that combined key demand-side interventions to reduce the cost of care at the point of use with supply-side interventions. The authors find that health care utilization in general was not undermined by the program, but some of the results using household data suggest there might have even been a negative impact on service use.

Second, the results confirm that the impact of UHC programs on utilization is usually heterogeneous and varies considerably, depending on factors such as population group (demographic and socioeconomic), regions covered, context specificities, program design, and time lag between the introduction of the intervention and the measurement of results. The most frequently analyzed source of heterogeneity is the changing impact across socioeconomic groups; in this case, several studies find that the worse-off seem to reap greater benefits in terms of access.

For example, Askeskin in Indonesia increases utilization of public care for the poorest quartile but there seems to be no impact for the richest (Sparrow, Suryahadi, and Widyanti 2013). Similarly, Cuevas and Parker (2011) find that health insurance in Indonesia increases outpatient and inpatient care utilization, but the size of the impact is greater on lower-income groups, and to some extent, also in rural areas. Gruber, Hendren, and Townsend (2012) find that the impact of the 30-Baht program in Thailand is greater among those previously enrolled in the Medical Welfare Scheme (MWS), a preexisting program that provided free care to low-income households and concentrated on a large fraction of the poorest now enrolled in the 30-Baht program. Panpiemras et al. (2011) report that the impact of the 30-Baht program in outpatient utilization tends to be higher in areas with lower average incomes.

Third, most UHC programs cannot be classified as simply "having" or "not having" an impact. Most studies' results show a "mixed" impact with positive impacts for some outcomes indicators but no impact for others. For example, several studies report positive impacts in utilization of out-patient visits but no significant effect on inpatient care (Miller, Pinto, and Vera-Hernández 2009; Powell-Jackson et al. 2014; Yip, Wang, and Hsiao 2008). Panpiemras et al. (2011) report that the 30-Baht program in Thailand increased outpatient visits, but they also find that the number of inpatient visits and the number of days for which the inpatients were admitted at hospitals actually declined.

Similarly, many studies that report overall favorable effects on access do not find a positive effect in every indicator analyzed. In addition, two studies that report no effect in access can still find positive effects in selected indicators. Johar (2009), for example, finds an increase in utiliza-tion of contraceptives among females eligible for a health card program targeted at the poor in Indonesia, but no effect on utilization of other services. Similarly, Wagstaff and Yu (2007) find that health care utiliza-tion in general was not impacted by the program, but they report positive impacts on the use of specific services (hepatitis B immunization and the incidence of nontesting of suspected TB patients).

Fourth, the relationship is complex between the interventions and the choice of health care source. Gruber, Hendren, and Townsend (2012) find that Thailand's Universal Health Care Coverage Program not only increased health care utilization overall but also led to a shift from public to private utilization among the previously uninsured. Powell-Jackson et al. (2014) report that an experiment on removing user fees in Ghana shifted care seeking away from informal providers. Yip, Wang, and Hsiao (2008) report that China's Rural Mutual Health Care (RMHC) increased outpatient visits and reduced self-medication to similar degrees. Micro health insurance in Cambodia increased the use of public health facilities covered by the program while reducing the use of other sources of care (Levine, Polimeni, and Ramage 2012). Similarly, Thornton et al. (2010) report that social security for the informal sector in Nicaragua led to a substitution of the source of health care toward the facilities covered by the program. Barros (2011) also reports a shift in the source of health care, from private to public, in the case of Mexico's Seguro Popular.

Finally, as other authors have argued (Acharya et al. 2013), higher health care *consumption* is not necessarily a welfare improvement, although most authors in the literature reviewed seem to agree that increased utilization is welfare-improving, given the relatively high levels of unmet health care needs in the countries analyzed (Miller, Pinto, and Vera-Hernández 2009, for example). There are, however, some excep-tions: Dourado et al. (2011) focus on the impact of Brazil's Family Health

Program (FHP) on hospital admissions for a set of primary care–sensitive conditions and they find that greater coverage leads to fewer hospital admissions for the selected conditions. This is presented as a favorable impact of the program that would be explained by improved access to timely and high-quality PHC that reduced the need for hospital care.

Overall, the evidence indicates that UHC programs, such as the ones evaluated in the literature reviewed, can indeed improve people's access to health care, but it also shows that the programs do not always work, do not work for everything, and do not affect everyone in the same way. Yet the role of the multiple factors conditioning the impact of the programs has not been regularly examined in the literature. Only one dimension has (changing impact across socioeconomic groups) and, although the results coincide in many cases (the worse-off seem to reap greater benefits), there are counterexamples (Wagstaff et al. 2009; Yip, Wang, and Hsiao 2008) that illustrate the difficulties of establishing an unequivocal relationship between UHC programs and outcomes.

The literature shows the potential of the evaluated UHC programs to help the countries advance toward UHC, but fails to understand thoroughly the complexities in the programs' causal chain and therefore provides little guidance for successful implementation beyond the contexts in which the programs have been originally put into practice.

Financial Protection—Impacts Are Mixed, and More Research Is Needed into the Key Factors Influencing Results

The majority of studies examining the impact of UHC programs on financial protection use OOPE as the main outcome indicator. Some articles also use measures such as catastrophic payments or impoverishment expenses that are based on OOPE; other studies analyze financial protection outcome beyond OOPE, by for example, analyzing asset accumulation, health-related debt, and changes in nonhealth consumption.

A number of studies report significant reductions in OOPE and related measures. For example, Nguyen et al. (2012) report that the Bangladesh voucher program considerably cut the amount paid for maternal health services. Levine, Polimeni, and Ramage (2012) find that micro-health insurance in Cambodia reduces the OOPE associated with serious health shocks. Several studies also report reductions in OOPE brought about by different health insurance programs in Vietnam (Nguyen 2012a; Wagstaff and Pradhan 2005; Wagstaff 2010). Miller, Pinto, and Vera-Hernández (2009) conclude that the Subsidized Regime in Colombia lowers health care expenses—particularly for inpatient services—and the probability of high expenses. Wagstaff and Yu (2007) find that the World Bank's Health VIII project in Gansu province, China, reduced OOPE and the incidence of catastrophic expenditure and impoverishment. Yip and Hsiao (2009) show that the RMHC program in China reduced impoverishment and that it is more effective than more traditional NCMS implementation approaches that combine medical savings accounts for outpatient care with insurance for catastrophic hospital expenditures. Babiarz et al. (2010) report that China's NCMS reduces OOPE.

A few studies examine the impact on indicators beyond OOPE and many—certainly not all—find favorable effects. Parmar et al. (2011) find that CBHI in Burkina Faso protects household assets, enabling accumulation and preventing households from selling assets due to health shocks. Wagstaff and Pradhan (2005) try to understand whether health insurance in Vietnam helps to reduce the impact of illness on households' actual consumption patterns and they find that the program reduced OOPE and increased nonmedical consumption. The size of the effect on nonmedical consumption seems larger than that on medical consumption, suggesting that the protective effect of the program operated not only through lower OOPE but also through reduced risk exposure that allows (risk-averse) households to stop "holding back" consumption to eventually cope with large OOPE.

Levine, Polimeni, and Ramage (2012) show that households enrolled in micro health insurance in Cambodia are less likely to take out a loan with interest, have lower debts, and are less likely to sell assets and land following a health shock. Powell-Jackson et al. (2014) find that removing user fees in Ghana reduces the probability of households having to borrow to pay for health care. Miller, Pinto, and Vera-Hernández (2009) report that the Subsidized Regime in Colombia reduces OOPE but do not find evidence that the program has any effect on expenditures on durable goods, household education, or consumption.

There are also several studies that find no or very weak effects of the UHC programs on financial protection indicators. Lei and Lin (2009) find no effect of the NCMS on OOPE in the previous four weeks. Nguyen (2012b) concludes that voluntary health insurance in Vietnam does not seem to impact OOPE (neither for outpatient nor for inpatient care). Thornton et al. (2010) find that, overall, there is no reduction in OOPE associated with social security health insurance in Nicaragua, although there seems to be a reduction in expenditures for laboratory tests.

Finally, a number of studies show evidence of programs increasing financial risk. Sparrow, Suryahadi, and Widyanti (2013) find that the Askeskin-subsidized SHI program targeted at the informal sector and the poor in Indonesia increases OOPE, the budget shares spent on health-related OOPE, and perhaps also the incidence of catastrophic spending. Wagstaff et al. (2009) find that the NCMS had no statistically significant effect on average OOPE but the evidence suggests that the program may have increased the cost per inpatient episode and the incidence of catastrophic payments for some households. Wagstaff and Lindelow (2008) analyze the impact of having any health insurance in China and although the results vary, the evidence suggests that health insurance in China increases rather than reduces OOPE and the risk of catastrophic and large expenses.

Overall, the evidence on financial protection is mixed. Results indicate that several programs have proven successful in providing financial protection to households, at least partially. However, many studies also show much weaker results and sometimes even negative impacts. But the reasons for failure or success are unclear, although some studies shed some light on the issue. For example, some indicate that increases in utilization may explain why OOPE does not fall due to the programs—e.g., Wagstaff et al. (2009)—but not all studies examine the link between access and financial protection variables. Other studies highlight issues related to design and implementation of the programs that may explain weak results, such as the appropriateness of the benefit package to the health care needs of the population. But here, too, as the key factors influencing the (positive or negative) results are rarely examined, there is not enough evidence to fully understand why rather similar interventions sometimes work, but sometimes fail to protect households against the financial risks of illness.

Health Status—Tentative Claims Can Be Made for Beneficial Impacts, but the Complex Chain of Causality Needs More Research

Similarly, the evidence on the impact of UHC programs on health status is mixed and there are no clear patterns that enable us to draw more general conclusions. On the one hand, several studies show little or no impact on health status indicators. Levine, Polimeni, and Ramage (2012) find that micro health insurance in Cambodia does not seem to affect the likelihood of individuals having serious health shocks, nor other indicators such as body mass index and height-for-age and weight-for-age. Chen and Jin (2010) and Lei and Lin (2009) do not find health improvements in health status associated with China's NCMS (they analyzed mortality of young children and pregnant women, self-reported health status, and sickness/injury in the four weeks preceding the survey). Cuevas and Parker (2011) analyze the impact of health insurance in Indonesia on several health outcome indicators and find little relationship between outcomes and the program. The evidence for Seguro Popular in Mexico also indicates that the implementation of the program has neither affected self-perceived health status nor other measures—arguably objective—such as incidence of health problems in general, the Activities for Daily Living disability index, and the prevalence of hypertension among adults (Barros 2011; King et al. 2009).

On the other hand, several examples illustrate that UHC programs *can* improve people's health. Quimbo et al. (2010) evaluate the impact of health insurance expansion in the Philippines and show that it decreases the likelihood of a sick child (with pneumonia or diarrhea) being wasted. The intervention shows no immediate impact on upon-discharge outcomes but only a few weeks later, suggesting that better health outcomes are not the result of higher quality of inpatient care but the result of other channels, such as improved financial protection due to insurance that allows households to afford supplementary medicines, increase food consumption, or improve access to outpatient care. Several studies examine the impact of Brazil's FHP and they all agree that higher coverage of the program is associated with reduced mortality (Aquino, de Oliveira, and Barreto 2009; Macinko, Guanais, and de Souza 2006; Rasella, Aquino, and Barreto 2010; Rocha and Soares 2010). Wagstaff and Pradhan (2005) find that Vietnam's health insurance program had a positive impact on height-for-age and weight-for-age of young school children, and on body mass index among adults. Plan Nacer in Argentina seems to increase birth weight, reduce the probability of very low birth weight, significantly improve newborn Apgar scores, and reduce the newborn early mortality rate (Gertler, Martinez, and Celhay 2011).

Beyond these mixed results, several studies are inconclusive due to methodological challenges. An interesting example of the importance of the selection of outcome indicators and sources of information for measurement come from Colombia's Subsidized Regime. Giedion, Diaz, and Alfonso (2007) use DHS surveys to measure child mortality, low birth weight, and self-perceived health status. The results indicate mostly no effect or a very weak effect of the program. The authors conclude that although there seems to be a program impact, the evidence is not conclusive and suggest that future research should focus on health outcomes more likely to be affected by the program and on better sources of information for measuring them. Camacho and Conover (2013) also evaluate the impact of the Subsidized Regime, but using administrative birth record data, which, they argue, are more appropriate because the information on newborn health is recorded by a health professional at the time of delivery, obviating their need to rely on parents' recall of information several years earlier (as in DHS surveys). In this case, the authors find that the Subsidized Regime appears to have lowered the incidence of low birth weight and to have had no detectable impact on other indicators, such as incidence of preterm deliveries, and higher five-minute Apgar scores.

The causality chain in the case of health status is even more complex than for access and financial protection. Methodological challenges are also greater. Hence, it is not surprising that several studies interpret weak results as inconclusive evidence rather than as failure. And although the evidence is neither extensive enough nor consistent enough to draw general conclusions, several examples indeed show that UHC programs can have a favorable impact on people's health. Further, although most authors seem to agree that the main pathway for the impact on health status is improved access to high-quality health care, other channels that may initially seem unlikely may be at work, as the example from the Philippines suggests. Once again, the evidence is insufficient to understand the complex causal chain behind the impacts of the UHC programs on health status.

A Synopsis of Some Other Literature Reviews

The search strategy also picked up related literature reviews. Ekman (2004) reviewed 16 studies that quantitatively examined the impact of CBHI and concludes that such arrangements can reduce OOPE and increase health care utilization. However, the size of the effect varies from study to study, and is sometimes rather small. Further, the initiatives evaluated faced challenges, such as sustainability, limited coverage, and targeting difficulties, that cast doubt on the actual ability of CBHI to provide financial protection and improve access to health care for many people. The author also remarks that the evidence is limited in scope, of questionable quality for internal validity, and not very useful for generalizations.

Meyer et al. (2011) reviewed 24 studies that evaluated 16 health voucher programs designed to reach specific populations and facilitate the use of selected health care services (for reproductive health and insecticide-treated bed nets; only one program for general health services). Overall, the authors find that health voucher programs seem to have increased the use of the selected services and that the literature does not show an evident link between the programs and the population's health. They also underscore that the evidence is insufficient to draw strong conclusions, particularly for the link with health outcomes. In addition, the review does not provide any insight on the "lessons learned" in implementing these programs.

Finally, several studies picked up in the review cannot provide a reliable estimate of the effect of the programs. Bellows, Bellows, and Warren (2011) reviewed literature on the use of vouchers for reproductive health services in developing countries with somewhat similar findings: voucher programs seem to be associated with increases in the utilization of reproductive health services, and *some* of them have improved health outcomes. However, once again, the authors conclude that more robustly designed studies are needed to more reliably establish a causal link between voucher programs and health care utilization and health outcomes.

Lagarde and Palmer (2011) reviewed 26 studies that examined the effect of introducing, removing, or changing user fees on health care utilization, health expenditures, or health outcomes. The results are mixed but generally suggest that when user fees are introduced or increased, health care utilization drops significantly. Conversely, when user fees are reduced or removed, the use of health care tends to increase, particularly for outpatient care and, after a while, for preventive services as well. The effects, however, vary considerably and the conclusions cannot therefore be regarded as definitive. The review found no effects of changing user fees on health expenditures or on health outcomes. The authors highlight that most studies have methodological weaknesses that suggest a high risk of bias, which, exacerbated by the variability of results, indicates that the evidence is highly uncertain.

Several reviews looked into the impact of programs called health insurance. Spaan et al. (2012) reviewed literature on the impact of health insurance in Africa and Asia, and they conclude that "there is, however, strong evidence that CBHI and SHI provide financial protection for their members in terms of reducing their OOPE, and that they improve utilization of inpatient and outpatient services" (Spaan et al. 2012, 687). However, the authors warn that the majority of studies relied on observational analysis that cannot reliably support causal inference. They also suggest that the results should be treated with caution given that the impact depends critically on the socioeconomic, cultural, and political context in which the programs are implemented.

Moreno-Serra and Smith (2012) reviewed the most robust cross-country studies examining the causal link between expansion in coverage and health outcomes, using extended risk pooling and prepayment as key indicators of progress toward universal coverage. They conclude that expansion in coverage normally leads to better population outcomes and that the health gains tend to be greater in poorer countries and among the poorest within countries. However, they highlight that the size of the impact varies greatly depending on context, characteristics of the population, institutional factors, and other variables for which researchers rarely have data on which to conduct a more thorough investigation, and recommend that these major data and methodological limitations should be tackled by research to better understand both the link between coverage and health outcomes and the specific factors driving the effectiveness (or lack thereof) of UHC efforts.

Acharya et al. (2013) reviewed literature on the impact of health insurance for the informal sector in low- and middle-income countries. The authors conclude that there is no strong evidence of an impact on utilization because only nine of 15 studies report higher utilization as a result of health insurance, and in some cases different results are obtained for the same program. Similarly, they report mainly mixed results for OOPE and health outcomes, indicating that "for most of the health insurance schemes, the poorest among the insured fared less well." The authors highlight the need to strengthen outcome measurements and evaluation methodologies in future studies, and to analyze further the pathways through which programs affect outcomes.

The reviews vary substantially in objectives, scope, search strategy, inclusion criteria, etc. and, thus, they are not directly comparable, but taken together leave a few messages that seem to be common. First, the quality of the evidence is often poor. Second, the evidence is sparse and insufficient to understand the effectiveness of a wide range of interventions being implemented. Third, studies do not always examine important sources of impact heterogeneity. Fourth, studies that attempt to establish a causal relationship frequently fail to understand the different links in the causal chain. In short, it would seem that the evidence base has to be strengthened.

Thoughts on the Strengths, Limitations, and Usefulness of Evidence for Policy Advice

Given the search strategy and inclusion criteria, the most salient strength of the studies included in the review is that they applied methods to establish a causal relationship between the UHC program and outcomes. This is very important because it allows analysts to identify "what works" to achieve the goals of the programs, making sure the changes are due to the interventions and not due to other potentially confounding factors. However, and perhaps paradoxically, most of the limitations are to some extent related to the constraints imposed by the methodological approach needed to rigorously estimate the causal effect of the interventions.

First, impact evaluations require a comparison group to mimic a counterfactual situation. For within-country evaluations such as those included in the review, this implies that evaluations compare two groups within a country (UHC program members vs. nonmembers, covered regions vs. not covered, etc.) to estimate the causal effect of the UHC program. This, however, may not be the right unit of analysis to understand the advances toward UHC because, frequently, it does not establish the contribution of the program on the UHC strategy as a whole (Kutzin 2013).

Second, and closely related, a major limitation of the studies reviewed is that most of them do not assess the potential spillover effects of the UHC programs evaluated. Only a couple of studies attempt to determine whether the UHC program had effects beyond the beneficiaries and other directly affected stakeholders, and all of them provide evidence of such effects (Babiarz et al. 2010; Yip, Wang, and Hsiao 2008). Measuring spillover effects is important because it not only helps to remove the bias from the estimates of the direct effects of the treatment but also provides a measure of the indirect effects, which is important for policy purposes and to avoid misleading guidance (Gertler et al. 2010; Khandker, Koolwal, and Samad 2009; White 2009). The UHC programs usually involve large interventions that may affect every component of the health system, which suggests that spillover effects may be pervasive for the UHC programs that are a key part of a broader UHC strategy. Addressing spillover effects would be a helpful step to shift the unit of analysis from the UHC program to a system-level analysis more consistent with UHC.

The problems above are compounded by the fact that usually those who do not benefit from the UHC program still have some form of coverage. Not being formally enrolled in a program is rarely equivalent to total lack of coverage as most countries offer basic coverage provided by a ministry of health. This misunderstanding may lead to confusing conclusions, misleading policy advice, or both.

The selection of outcome indicators is sometimes a limitation of the studies reviewed. For example, a few studies rely only on indicators such as number of visits, and that may be problematic because they may overlook those who do not seek care at all. Similarly, traditional measures of financial protection based on OOPE have been recently criticized for being a narrow view of a very complex problem, and several studies rely only on OOPE. Major concerns are that the measures: fail to capture cost barriers to access, and hence categorize those who cannot afford care as spending little or nothing on care and so erroneously classify them as financially protected; frequently do not include other health-seeking related costs beyond direct payments, such as transportation costs or informal (under-the-table) payments; do not capture other strategies to cope with costs of illness such as reduced household consumption of other goods and services or increasing debt to finance health expenses; and do not include indirect costs such as income loss due to illness (Lu et al. 2009; Moreno-Serra, Millett, and Smith 2011; Ruger 2012; Wagstaff 2008).

Finally, perhaps the biggest limitation of this research is that it provides little insight on the pathways and mechanisms at work for UHC programs to affect outcomes. The evaluations show *which* UHC programs have a favorable impact on outcomes, but not *why* a specific program succeeds or fails to improve outcomes. Only a few studies provide direct evidence on the individual contribution of specific program components to program impact—see, for example, Wagstaff et al. (2009) and Yip, Wang, and Hsiao (2008). Also, only a small number of studies provide additional evidence on the key contextual factors enabling (or hindering) success.

The majority of studies provide little insight on how the design, implementation, or context of the UHC programs conditioned their effectiveness, and no or very little evidence on the different steps of the causal chain between the UHC programs and outcomes. This is a major drawback because it diminishes the usefulness of the evidence to inform policy. To design and implement a UHC program, decision makers face myriad policy options in several program components. To navigate such complexity, studies that simply determine whether a multifaceted program affected some outcome indicators may not be very useful.

TABLE C.1
Summary of Findings by Program

Country, health coverage program, and authors	Summary of findings
Argentina—Plan Nacer (Gertler, Martinez, and Celhay 2011)	*Access:* Plan Nacer increases early detection of pregnant women by 2.5 and 4.9 percentage points, for visits before the 13th and 20th week of pregnancy, respectively. The program reduces the probability of the first visit after the 20th week of pregnancy by 7.4 percentage points. The program also increases the number of prenatal care visits by 0.5 visits on average, which represents a 16% rise. In addition, the program also increases the probability of healthy-child checkups according to guidelines: a 32.7% rise for children 45–70 days old, 21.5% 70–120 days, and 18.2% 120–200 days, but no significant effect for children over 200 days old. *Health status:* Plan Nacer increased birth weight by 2% (69.5 g), reduced the probability of very low birth weight by 26%, and brought significant, albeit modest, improvements in newborn Apgar scores. Plan Nacer also reduced the newborn early mortality rate by 1.9 percentage points.
Bangladesh—Bangladesh Voucher Program (Nguyen et al. 2012)	*Access:* The voucher program provides free access to selected maternal and child health care services as well as coverage for transport costs, a gift box (worth US$7.29), and a cash incentive after delivering with a qualified provider. Results show a positive impact of the program in health care-seeking behavior from qualified providers (for antenatal care, delivery, and postnatal care) and an increase in institutional delivery. However, no significant effect of the program was observed on the rate of deliveries by cesarean section. *Financial protection:* The authors find that women in program intervention areas are less likely to incur out-of-pocket expenditures (OOPE) and that they also paid approximately Taka 640 (US$9.43) less for maternal health care services, equivalent to 64% of the sample's average monthly household expenditure per capita.

table continues next page

TABLE C.1 *(Continued)*

Country, health coverage program, and authors	Summary of findings
Brazil—Family Health Program (Aquino, de Oliveira, and Barreto 2009)	*Health status:* Higher coverage levels of the Family Health Program (FHP) is associated with reductions in infant mortality rates at the municipality level. Relative to municipalities with no coverage of the program, on average, low coverage (incipient) reduces infant mortality by 13%, intermediate coverage by 16%, and a consolidated FHP by 22%. The effect is greater on post-neonatal mortality (18%, 22%, 31%) than on neonatal mortality (10%, 14%, 19%). In addition, the effect of the program is greater in municipalities with higher mortality rates and those with a lower human development index.
Brazil—Family Health Program (Dourado et al. 2011)	*Access:* Using data at the state level, the authors find that greater coverage of the FHP is associated with reduced hospital admissions for Primary Health Care Sensitive Conditions (PHCSC). PHCSC are a set of conditions that can reasonably be prevented by timely access to high-quality PHC. The authors report that higher coverage of the FHP is associated with at least 5% reduction in hospital PHCSC admissions. Although the authors do not have the data to be certain that it was FHP users who had lower PHCSC admissions, the evidence suggests that the FHP reduced hospitalization needs by improving access to primary care and perhaps by improving people's health.
Brazil—Family Health Program (Macinko, Guanais, and de Souza 2006)	*Health status:* Using data at the level of federative units, the authors find that higher coverage of the FHP is associated with lower infant mortality. On average, given the levels of coverage in the period 1990–2002, a 10% increase in coverage of the program is associated with a 4.6% reduction in infant mortality.
Brazil—Family Health Program (Rasella, Aquino, and Barreto 2010)	*Health status:* Higher coverage of the FHP is associated with reductions in under-five mortality rates at the municipality level. The effect is greater for unattended death (26%, 43%, 60% reductions for low, intermediate, and high coverage) than for mortality due to ill-defined causes (17%, 35%, 50%).
Brazil—Family Health Program (Rocha and Soares 2010)	*Health status:* The authors find that the FHP reduces mortality. The effect is particularly strong on infant mortality, but it holds for other age groups. The size of the effect changes with the time of exposure to the program; for example, for municipalities that have been three years in the program, the mortality rate for children between their first birthday and the day before their fifth birthday decreases by 6.7% and the impact in municipalities with eight years in the program is a 24% reduction in mortality. In addition, the poorest regions of the country and the municipalities with worse initial conditions reap greater benefits from the program. Consistent with the program's intervention, the largest impacts are associated with mortality due to perinatal period conditions, infectious diseases, influenza, asthma, and bronchitis.
Burkina Faso—Community-based health insurance (Gnawali et al. 2009)	*Access:* The authors find a positive impact of community-based health insurance (CBHI) on outpatient visits for those who are ill (increase of nearly 40% among those enrolled) but no detectable effect on the use of inpatient care. Among those enrolled, the very poor remain less likely to use health care services.

table continues next page

TABLE C.1 *(Continued)*

Country, health coverage program, and authors	Summary of findings
Burkina Faso—Community-based health insurance (Parmar et al. 2011)	*Financial protection:* CBHI in rural areas was shown to have a financial protection effect of a 1–24.6% increase in per capita household assets. Its maximum protective effect might have coincided with an economic downturn in the area and a spike in illness. The authors hypothesize that the observed increase in wealth may have been the result of the protective effect of CBHI through two channels: beneficiaries avoid selling productive assets (livestock); and beneficiaries receive highly subsidized premiums.
Burkina Faso—Community-based health insurance (Robyn et al. 2012)	*Access:* Results show that CBHI introduced in Nouna health district had no effect on health-seeking behavior. The authors examined the effect of the program on the health-seeking behavior of individuals reporting a health problem in the 30 days preceding the interview (health care seeking in general and treatment from facility-based professional care). The authors also discuss several reasons that may explain the weak results, including poor perceived quality of care, dissatisfaction with the program, and lack of understanding of the benefit package by enrollees as well as the payment methods for health care providers that may cause preferential treatment to the noninsured over the insured.
Cambodia—Micro-health insurance (Levine, Polimeni, and Ramage 2012)	*Access:* The authors find that health insurance (at deeply discounted price) did not substantially affect health care utilization; for most indicators there is usually no detectable effect or it is very small (although in some cases, such as preventive care, the sample has low statistical power to detect small effects). However, being insured did change health-seeking behavior by reducing the use of private providers as the first source of care by 11 percentage points and drug sellers by 8 percentage points, and increasing the use of public health centers by 18 percentage points. *Financial protection:* Insurance is found to reduce annual OOPE by 44%. Much of this saving is due to lower rates of high medical expenses. The financial protection brought by health insurance goes beyond lower OOPE: insured households are 9.2 percentage points less likely to sell assets following a health shock and 13.6 percentage points less likely to take out a loan at interest. Similarly, insured households have nearly 33% lower debts and are also 1.6 percentage points less likely to sell land for health reasons. *Health status:* The authors detect no effect on health status, in particular, no effect of insurance was found on the likelihood of individuals having a serious health shock, nor on further indicators such as body mass index, height-for-age, and weight-for-age.
China—Any health insurance scheme (Wagstaff and Lindelow 2008)	*Financial protection:* The authors analyze the impact of having any health insurance in China, using three different surveys that vary in geographic coverage (second-poorest province, central and eastern provinces, central and western provinces), and a rural-urban focus (two of them rural only, one urban and rural). Although the results vary considerably, the three surveys suggest that health insurance in China increases rather than reduces both OOPE and the risk of catastrophic and large expenses.
China—New Cooperative Medical Scheme (Babiarz et al. 2010)	*Access:* The authors find that the New Cooperative Medical Scheme (NCMS) has no detectable effect on the probability of individuals seeking medical care in case of illness. However, they find a change in the type of facility used; NCMS enrollees are 5% more likely to attend a village clinic and less likely to use township health centers or larger hospitals.

table continues next page

TABLE C.1 *(Continued)*

Country, health coverage program, and authors	Summary of findings
	This is somehow corroborated by the data at the facility level: the NCMS is associated with an increase in average weekly patient flow for village clinics eligible for reimbursement by the NCMS (26% increase) or simply being in a village with an NCMS program (55% increase). *Financial protection:* The authors find that participation in the NCMS is associated with a 19% reduction in total annual medical OOPE. In addition, the NCMS seems to lower the probability of incurring high expenditures and the likelihood of financing medical care through asset sales or borrowing.
China—New Cooperative Medical Scheme (Chen and Jin 2010)	*Health status:* Using a large census database, the authors find no effect of the NCMS on health status outcomes (mortality of young children and pregnant women). Although enrollees have on average better outcomes than nonenrollees, such a difference is explained by endogenous introduction and take-up of the program. After controlling for such effects, no impact is found. According to the authors, the lack of impact might be explained by the low reimbursement rate of the NCMS and the fact that mortality is an extreme event that is difficult to affect.
China—New Cooperative Medical Scheme (Lei and Lin 2009)	*Access:* The authors find that the NCMS increases the probability of using any preventive-care services in the last four weeks (by around 60–85%), driven mostly by access to general physical examinations and not other preventive care. The authors find no effect on the use of formal medical care, neither in all the sample nor among those who felt sick in the last four weeks. *Financial protection:* The authors find no effect of the NCMS on OOPE in the last four weeks. *Health status:* The authors find no overall effect of the program on health status measures (self-reported health status, sickness/injury within the four weeks preceding the survey). Only one of the specifications (PSM-DID) shows a small effect of the NCMS on the probability of feeling sick or injured (a decrease of 2.8 percentage points).
China—New Cooperative Medical Scheme (Wagstaff et al. 2009)	*Access:* Results indicate that the scheme has increased outpatient and inpatient utilization by 20 to 30%. No impact was found among the poorest. This result may be related to the fact that the budget is too small to make a significant difference in households' OOPE. The revenue per enrolled is around only one-fifth of total per capita rural health spending, and copayments in the scheme are high, reflecting large deductibles, low ceilings, and high coinsurance rates. The "affordability dimension" of access among the poorest may therefore be only slightly changed, the NCMS explaining why no impact was found in this group. *Financial protection:* The authors find that the NCMS has had no statistically significant effect on average OOPE by households overall or on any specific type of care per episode, for either outpatient or inpatient care. The analyses seem to suggest that the NCMS may have increased the cost per inpatient episode. Further, the NCMS appears to have increased the incidence of catastrophic household OOPE, at least where the catastrophic threshold is 20% or less of income.

table continues next page

TABLE C.1 *(Continued)*

Country, health coverage program, and authors	Summary of findings
China—New Cooperative Medical Scheme (Yip and Hsiao 2009)	*Financial protection:* The NCMS reduced the poverty headcount, average poverty gap, and positive poverty gap. Comparing the effect of the traditional model of the NCMS (based on medical savings accounts and a high-deductible catastrophic hospital insurance) with the Rural Mutual Health Care (RMHC) program (based on first dollar coverage with a similar premium as the NCMS but a lower ceiling), the RMHC is found to be more effective in reducing impoverishment.
China—Rural Mutual Health Care (Yip, Wang, and Hsiao 2008)	*Access:* The RMHC program has increased the probability of an outpatient visit by 70% and reduced the probability of self-medication by a similar proportion. The study also finds evidence of spillover effects in which no enrollees of the RMHC sites increased the probability of visits. The study further estimates the impacts of a variation of the NCMS that combines medical savings accounts and hospital insurance with high deductibles, finding little impact (no impact on inpatient utilization and a positive effect on outpatient care, but much weaker than that of RMHC). Finally, the authors find that affiliates belonging to the lowest- and highest-income strata experienced the greatest increase in outpatient visits to village doctors, whereas the middle-income group experienced the most important increase in utilization of health care services at township level.
China—Rural Mutual Health Care (Wang et al. 2009)	*Health status:* The results show that RMHC had a positive effect on the health status of participants. Among EQ-5D five dimensions (EQ-5D™ is a standardized instrument for use as a measure of health outcomes), RMHC significantly reduced pain/discomfort and anxiety/depression for the general population. Differences in the effect of RMHC on overall health outcomes stratified by income, gender, age, and illness status at baseline are found; lowest income groups experienced the greatest health improvement. Those who were "ill" in the baseline experienced a greater reduction in reporting any problem in EQ-5D. Those above 55 years benefited most in terms of improved mobility and continuing their usual activities.
China—World Bank's Health VIII project in Gansu province (Wagstaff and Yu 2007)	*Access:* The authors find mixed evidence on the impact of the project on the use of health care services. a small impact on utilization. They found no impact on some indicators such as outpatient visits or inpatient admissions and perhaps even a negative impact on doctor visits. Conversely, some indicators such as immunizations show a positive impact. *Financial protection:* The authors find that the project reduced OOPE, the incidence of catastrophic spending, and impoverishment from health expenses. The impact was especially important among the poorest. *Health status:* Results indicate the project may have reduced the number of days of sickness, at least among the poor (and among the third quintile) and chronic sickness for the poorest quintile. Results on self-assessed health are mixed and not robust across the various methods.
Colombia—Subsidized Regime (Camacho and Conover 2013)	*Access:* The authors find evidence suggesting that the Subsidized Regime may have increased the likelihood of giving birth at a hospital or health center. However, the program does not seem to change prenatal care visits or doctor-assisted deliveries indicators.

table continues next page

TABLE C.1 *(Continued)*

Country, health coverage program, and authors	Summary of findings
	Health status: The authors find that the Subsidized Regime appears to have lowered the incidence of low birth weight by 1.7–3.8 percentage points (16–36% of the total rate of low birth weight). No detectable impact was found in other indicators such as birth weight, incidence of very low birth weight, incidence of preterm deliveries, and higher five-minute Apgar scores (although the direction of the estimates shows a positive tendency in all of them—higher, lower, lower, higher, respectively).
Colombia—Subsidized Regime (Giedion, Diaz, and Alfonso 2007)	*Access:* Evidence from the different methodologies consistently indicates that the Subsidized Regime has considerably improved access and utilization of curative and preventive health care services. These gains have also been found for services free to all irrespective of an individual's insurance status, indicating that health insurance may not only have an impact through the affordability dimension of access. The impact has been especially important among rural and the poorest populations.
	Health status: No conclusive evidence is found. The study suggests the need to develop health status variables able to capture the more subtle kind of changes underlying quality of life that may result from improved access to health care services due to health insurance.
Colombia—Subsidized Regime (Miller, Pinto, and Vera-Hernández 2009)	*Access:* The authors find that the Subsidized Regime substantially increases the use of traditionally underutilized preventive services; the probability of a preventive physician visit in the past year increases by 29 percentage points and enrolled children have 1.24 more growth-monitoring and well-care visits in the past year. The use of curative medical care also seems to improve due to enrollment in the program: the probability of a visit to a physician because of health problems within the past 30 days increases by 13 percentage points. However, no effects are found on curative care among children, hospitalizations, or medical visits for chronic diseases.
	Financial protection: The authors find that the Subsidized Regime lowers mean inpatient spending by about 31%, reduces the variability of inpatient spending by 34%, and reduces the likelihood of high inpatient spending at different thresholds. Results also show that outpatient spending is not affected by enrollment in the program. Although results from OOPE suggest the program provides meaningful risk protection to households, it does not seem to affect broader measures of household finances: no detectable effects are found in the composition of household assets, human capital investments (education), and consumption expenditures.
	Health status: The authors examine the effect of the program on health status indicators that can be linked to increases in preventive service use. They find that enrollment is associated with 1.3 fewer child days absent from usual activities due to illness in the past month and a 35 percentage point reduction in the self-reported incidence of cough, fever, or diarrhea among children in the preceding two weeks (a 62% reduction).
Costa Rica—National health insurance (Dow and Schmeer 2003)	*Health status:* Insurance coverage increases are strongly related to mortality decreases at county level before controlling for other time-varying factors. However, after controlling for changes in other correlated maternal, household, and community characteristics, fixed-effects models indicate that the insurance expansion had a significant but only small impact on child mortality rates.

table continues next page

TABLE C.1 *(Continued)*

Country, health coverage program, and authors	Summary of findings
Georgia—Medical Insurance Program (Bauhoff, Hotchkiss, and Smith 2010)	*Access:* The evidence suggests that there was no impact of this program on utilization outcomes (neither inpatient nor outpatient care). However, an impact was identified on provider choices: beneficiaries increased their likelihood of using primary care facilities in some regions while reducing the likelihood of using pharmacies in others. The authors believe this result might be explained by obstacles in program implementation, that the main source of OOPE (pharmaceuticals) is not covered, the short implementation time, the perceived quality of care, or access restrictions imposed by insurance companies. *Financial protection:* Although the results vary across specifications and regions, the evidence seems to suggest that the program reduces outpatient OOPE, especially among the elderly. For inpatient care, there is clear evidence of a reduction in OOPE that are, for beneficiaries, about 42–60% of what nonbeneficiaries spend. It also considerably reduced the risk of high inpatient expenditures.
Georgia—Medical Insurance Program (Hou and Chao 2011)	*Access:* Results show that the program had a positive impact on the use of acute surgeries/inpatient care reimbursed by public health insurance schemes. The authors also show evidence that the benefits of the program have reached the poor because the lowest quintiles have a higher probability than the highest quintile of utilization of services reimbursed by the program.
Ghana—User fee removal (Powell-Jackson et al. 2014)	*Access:* The authors find that removing user fees led to increased utilization of primary health clinics (an increase of 0.3 visits per year or 12%) but no change in hospital visits. The results also show that the increase in PHC clinics utilization resulted mostly from a substitution from informal health care providers, given that removing user fees also led to a reduction in the use of informal care (0.28 fewer visits per year or 9% reduction). *Financial protection:* The authors find that the removal of user fees reduced OOPE in the past four weeks by 27%. It also reduced the likelihood of having to borrow to pay for health care in the last four weeks by 3.4 percentage points (40%). *Health status:* Removing user fees did not have any detectable effect on health status of the population. The authors examined the impact on several indicators, including anemia (level of hemoglobin in blood), malaria parasitemia, height-for-age, weight-for-age, and weight-for-height, and they found no significant effect on any of these indicators.
Indonesia—Askeskin (Sparrow, Suryahadi, and Widyanti 2013)	*Access:* The authors find that Askeskin—a subsidized social health insurance program targeted at the informal sector and the poor—has a favorable effect on overall utilization. Results indicate that the program increased outpatient utilization by 0.062 visits per person per month. This effect is mostly driven by a net increase in utilization of public health care providers (private sector utilization only seems to increase in urban areas). The results also show that the bulk increase in utilization occurred among the poorest as the effect is significant for the lowest quartile (and in some cases for the second-lowest quartile) while there seems to be no impact for the richest. *Financial protection:* The authors find that Askeskin seems to increase OOPE and the share of the budget spent on health OOPE. The bulk of the effect is seen in urban areas. In addition, and although the results vary, there is also some evidence of increased incidence of catastrophic spending. Thus the program seems to increase the financial risk presumably, according to the authors, because the insured had to bear part of the costs of increased health care utilization.

table continues next page

TABLE C.1 *(Continued)*

Country, health coverage program, and authors	Summary of findings
Indonesia—Health card program (Johar 2009)	*Access:* Overall, results indicate that the health card program had, if anything, a limited impact on the use of health care. The authors examined the effect of the program on the use of preventive and curative outpatient care as well as inpatient care in private and public facilities, and in most cases the results show no program effect. The authors only find detectable impacts of the program among children (a positive impact on the use of public health facilities for outpatient curative care) and for spouses (a shift of the source of care; and lower use of private providers for preventive care that seems to be largely driven by increased demand for contraception at public facilities).
Indonesia—Health Insurance (Askes, Asabri, Jamsostek) (Cuevas and Parker 2011)	*Access:* The authors find that having health insurance increases the probability of having any outpatient care in the four weeks prior to the survey (an increase of nearly 4 percentage points in urban areas and 5 percentage points in rural areas). Insurance also seems to increase the number of outpatient visits and the effect is slightly larger for the rural population, especially women. The results for inpatient care in the last 12 months also show positive effects of insurance, but only in rural areas. In addition, the worse off seem to reap greater benefits from the program; for example, the effect on the number of outpatient visits is nearly 2.5 times greater among adults in the bottom 50% of the expenditure distribution than those in the top 50% of the distribution. *Financial protection:* Insurance is found to reduce the probability of having any household health spending (by 3–5 percentage points). However, there seems to be no impact on average per capita health spending in the household. *Health status:* Many health status indicators show little relationship with insurance status, though a few seem to improve: a reduction of problems in daily activities for adults; a potential impact in reducing high blood pressure in adults for lower-income groups; and a reduction in child obesity in some groups (but an increase in others).
Indonesia—Safe Motherhood Project (Baird, Ma, and Ruger 2011)	*Health status:* The authors find no detectable effects of the program on indicators such as infant mortality, total fertility rate, teenage pregnancy, unmet contraceptive need, or percentage of deliveries overseen by trained health personnel. However, the program seems to be associated with improvements in under-five mortality. Both intervention and control groups improved in several indicators, perhaps also due to the effect of two other concurrent development projects.
Mexico—Seguro Popular (Barros 2011)	*Access:* The author finds that the program did not cause an increase in the total demand for curative services by beneficiaries. The probability of seeking care when there is a health problem or the probability of not seeking care for financial reasons does not seem to have been affected by the program. However, the program seems to have caused a substitution from private to public providers. *Financial protection:* Results indicate that the program led to a large reduction in the probability of OOPE. Similarly, it reduces the probability of catastrophic expenditures. However, the program does not seem to considerably change the amount spent (although some results indicate there might have been a reduction in OOPE for curative care). Finally, the author finds a reduction in the household budget share for health but no change in total expenditure, implying that households used the resources freed by the program for consumption of other types of goods rather than savings.

table continues next page

TABLE C.1 *(Continued)*

Country, health coverage program, and authors	Summary of findings
	Health status: The author finds no detectable effect of the program in arguably objective measures of health status such as the incidence of health problems in general, the activities of daily living disability index, and the prevalence of hypertension among adults. However, the results indicate that the program seems to improve people's perception of their own health, shifting from poor and fair health to good health.
Mexico—Seguro Popular (King et al. 2009)	*Access:* No significant effect was found on the use of medical services, even though a wide range of measures was used. Further, subgroup analyses for low-asset, high-asset, and female-headed households were carried out and showed no significant effects. These results, however, do not mean that the program did not (and cannot) increase utilization, but only that such effects did not arise in the short assessment period (10 months).
	Financial protection: The program reduces the proportion of catastrophic health expenditures by 23–55%, and most of this effect occurs in low-asset households. It also reduces OOPE for all services, particularly for low-asset households. The reduction in expenditures is especially noticeable for inpatient and outpatient medical care, although no impact was found on medicines and medical devices. The authors hypothesize that the fact that no effect was found on OOPE for medicines and medical devices might be explained by the short assessment period (10 months); although price reduction for inpatient and outpatient care is immediate, the delivery of medicines might require a longer implementation period since it involves more complex administrative processes (like open bids for purchasing medicines).
	Health status: Although a positive effect seems to have initially occurred, further examination of the baseline data using difference-in-differences analysis demonstrates that such positive effect was mostly a placebo effect that appeared even in the baseline, and correcting for this reveals a small and close-to-zero effect.
Nicaragua—Social security health insurance for the informal sector (Thornton et al. 2010)	*Access:* Findings show that insurance does not increase the probability of seeking care overall, nor does it increase the number of visits. However, it creates a substitution effect in both indicators, driving care-seeking behavior from public and private facilities to empaneled facilities covered by the insurance.
	Financial protection: There is no overall reduction in OOPE, but there is a reduction in expenditures on laboratory tests.
Philippines—Health Insurance (QIDS experiment)—PhilHealth (Kraft et al. 2009)	*Access:* The authors find an impact of the insurance scheme in an increase in the number of children whose hospital care is not delayed.
Philippines—Health Insurance (QIDS experiment)—PhilHealth (Quimbo et al. 2010)	*Health status:* The intervention decreases the likelihood of a child being CRP-positive or wasted by 4 and 9 percentage points, respectively, for post-discharge outcomes. However, the intervention shows no immediate impact on on-discharge outcomes, suggesting that better health outcomes are not the result of higher quality of inpatient care; rather, other channels may operate such as improved financial protection brought by insurance that allows households to afford supplementary medicines, increase food consumption, or improve access to outpatient care.

table continues next page

TABLE C.1 *(Continued)*

Country, health coverage program, and authors	Summary of findings
Thailand—Universal Health Care Coverage (30 Baht program) (Gruber, Hendren, and Townsend 2012)	*Access:* The authors find that the 30 Baht program led to increased health care utilization. The estimates indicate that the program increased by 12% inpatient utilization among those previously enrolled in the Medical Welfare Scheme (MWS) and had a more modest effect on the previously uninsured (an increase of 8% over the baseline utilization). Consistent with the program design to provide free care only in public facilities, the results show a substitution of the source of care: an increase in utilization of public facilities and a decrease of private utilization. In addition, the impact of the program is stronger for women aged 20–30 years and infants, particularly among those previously enrolled in the MWS. *Health status:* The authors find that the 30 Baht program led to a reduction in infant mortality for the MWS group of at least 6.45 per 1,000 births, corresponding to an aggregate reduction in the national infant mortality rate of at least 2 per 1,000 births. The result is quite robust to several specifications; in particular, the authors provide evidence to support the claim that the results are not driven by changes in vital statistics recording around the introduction of the 30 Baht program or other contemporaneous factors correlated with the fraction of MWS enrollees in each province.
Thailand—Universal Health Care Coverage (30 Baht program) (Panpiemras et al. 2011)	*Access:* The authors found that the program increased outpatient demand for health care, particularly among the elderly and the poor. This increase, however, was strong in the first year of the program and faded in subsequent years. Conversely, the authors find a decline in inpatient visits.
Vietnam—Children's health insurance (free school health insurance, free preschool health insurance, Health Care Fund for the Poor) (Nguyen 2012a)	*Access:* The authors find that three health insurance programs (two specifically for children) do not influence outpatient utilization. They examined the effect on the number of annual outpatient contacts and the results indicate that neither school health insurance nor the free health insurance program has a significant impact. The impact on inpatient care was not examined because only a few children in the data set reported use of inpatient care. *Financial protection:* The authors examined the impact of two health insurance programs for children (free school health insurance and free preschool health insurance) on OOPE per outpatient contact. Results indicate that both programs seem to decrease the OOPE per outpatient contact (by 14% and 26%, respectively).
Vietnam—Voluntary health insurance (Nguyen 2012b)	*Access:* The authors find that voluntary health insurance has a positive impact on health care utilization, increasing the average number of annual visits by around 45% (outpatient) and nearly 70% (inpatient). The effect is similar across people with different health insurance status in 2004 as well as those who have been continuing to be insured since the previous period and those newly insured in the current period. *Financial protection:* Voluntary health insurance does not seem to have an impact on OOPE (outpatient or inpatient). The authors suggest that this result may be explained by the measure of OOPE used that includes not only the treatment fee but also all costs related to the treatment such as bonus for doctors, service charge for additional medicine requirements, equipment, and transportation.

table continues next page

TABLE C.1 *(Continued)*

Country, health coverage program, and authors	Summary of findings
Vietnam—Health Care Fund for the Poor (Wagstaff 2010)	*Access:* The health insurance program for poor households (Health Care Fund for the Poor) does not seem to change utilization of health care. *Financial protection:* The evidence shows that the program reduces considerably OOPE for outpatient and inpatient care.
Vietnam—Vietnam Health Insurance (Wagstaff and Pradhan 2005)	*Financial protection:* Results indicate that the program covering (at the time) mainly formal sector workers caused a reduction in annual OOPE on health, and an increase in nonmedical household consumption, mainly nonfood. *Health status:* The program influenced favorably the height-for-age and weight-for-age of young school children. It had a significant impact on the body mass index of adults, which rises monotonically with per capita household consumption, and as with weight-for-age among young children, there is no evidence of any beneficial effect of the program on nutritional status among the poorest quintile.

Notes

1. We excluded the following types of interventions: conditional cash transfer (CCT) programs, experiences with community health workers (CHW) for specific diseases (e.g., malaria), and initiatives focusing on goods rather than health care services (e.g., insecticide-treated bed nets).
2. We included in the list Universal Health Coverage Studies Series (UNICO) UHC programs, other programs mentioned in articles discussing the UHC movement, and other sources (UHC Forward Initiative, Joint Learning Network).
3. It comprises methods based on randomized selection, regression discontinuity designs, differences-in-differences (we also included fixed-effects and triple differencing models), and matching.
4. For example, a randomized promotion used as IV or the use of the placement in a cluster randomized trial with imperfect compliance as IV to estimate the treatment on the treated rather than the intention to treat.
5. PubMed, Econlit, EconBase (Elsevier), Ingenta, Social Science Research Network, ProQuest, Cambridge journals database, Jstor, Oxford journals database, Science Direct, Springerlink, Wiley Online.
6. The Brookings Institution, the World Bank, the World Health Organization (WHO), the Inter-American Development Bank, the Joint Learning Network, the International Initiative for Impact Evaluation (3IE), the Campbell Collaboration, and Google Scholar.
7. Universal coverage, UHC, health program, health programme, health coverage programme, universal access scheme, health intervention, health scheme, health insurance, community-based health insurance, community health insurance, CBHI, social health insurance, SHI, voucher, mutuelle, health card, coupon.

8. Access, accessibility, utilization, use of health care, financial protection, catastrophic health expenditure, catastrophic health payments, out-of-pocket expenditures (OOPE), out-of-pocket payments, private payments, direct payments, copayments, impoverishment, health status, health outcomes.
9. Impact, effect, consequence, evaluation, quantitative methods, results, differences in differences, double differences, regression discontinuity, randomized, experimental.

References

Acharya, A., S. Vellakkal, F. Taylor, E. Massett, A. Satija, M. Burke, and S. Ebrahim. 2013. "The Impact of Health Insurance Schemes for the Informal Sector in Low- and Middle-Income Countries: A Systematic Review." Policy Research Working Paper 6324, World Bank, Washington, DC.

Aquino, R., N. F. de Oliveira, and M. L. Barreto. 2009. "Impact of the Family Health Program on Infant Mortality in Brazilian Municipalities." *American Journal of Public Health* 99 (1): 87.

Babiarz, K. S., G. Miller, H. Yi, L. Zhang, and S. Rozelle. 2010. "New Evidence on the Impact of China's New Rural Cooperative Medical Scheme and Its Implications for Rural Primary Healthcare: Multivariate Difference-in-Difference Analysis." *BMJ* 341. doi:10.1136/bmj.c5617.

Baird, J., S. Ma, and J. P. Ruger. 2011. "Effects of the World Bank's Maternal and Child Health Intervention on Indonesia's Poor: Evaluating the Safe Motherhood Project." *Social Science & Medicine* 72 (12): 1948–55. http://www.sciencedirect.com/science/article/pii/S0277953610003916.

Barros, R. 2011. "Wealthier but Not Much Healthier: Effects of a Health Insurance Program for the Poor in Mexico." Working Paper, Stanford University.

Bauhoff, S., D. Hotchkiss, and O. Smith. 2010. "The Impact of Medical Insurance for the Poor in Georgia: A Regression Discontinuity Approach." *Health Economics* (October). http://ssrn.com/paper=1790565.

Bellows, N. M., B. W. Bellows, and C. Warren. 2011. "Systematic Review: The Use of Vouchers for Reproductive Health Services in Developing Countries: Systematic Review." *Tropical Medicine & International Health* 16 (1): 84–96.

Camacho, A., and E. Conover. 2013. "Effects of Subsidized Health Insurance on Newborn Health in a Developing Country." *Economic Development and Cultural Change* 61 (3): 633–58. http://www.jstor.org/stable/10.1086/669263.

Chen, Y., and G. Z. Jin. 2010. "Does Health Insurance Coverage Lead to Better Health and Educational Outcomes? Evidence from Rural China." National Bureau of Economic Research Working Paper. http://www.nber.org/papers/w16417.pdf.

Cuevas, F., and S. W. Parker. 2011. "The Impact of Health Insurance on Use, Spending, and Health in Indonesia." In *The Impact of Health Insurance on Low- and Middle-Income Countries*, edited by M.-L. Escobar, 122–36. Washington, DC: Brookings Institution Press.

Dourado, I., V. B. Oliveira, R. Aquino, P. Bonolo, M. F. Lima-Costa, M. G. Medina, E. Mota, M. A. Turci, and J. Macinko. 2011. "Trends in Primary Health Care-Sensitive Conditions in Brazil: The Role of the Family Health Program (Project ICSAP-Brazil)." *Medical Care* 49 (6): 577–84.

Dow, W. H., and K. K. Schmeer. 2003. "Health Insurance and Child Mortality in Costa Rica." *Social Science & Medicine* 57 (6): 975–86. http://www.sciencedirect.com/science/article/pii/S0277953602004641.

Ekman, B. 2004. "Community-Based Health Insurance in Low-Income Countries: A Systematic Review of the Evidence." *Health Policy and Planning* 19 (5): 249–70. http://heapol.oxfordjournals.org/content/19/5/249.abstract.

Gertler, P. J., S. Martinez, and P. Celhay. 2011. *Impacto del programa plan nacer sobre utilizacion de servicios y resultados sanitarios: resultados con datos administrativos de las provincias de misiones y tucumán*. Washington DC: World Bank.

Gertler, P. J., S. Martinez, P. Premand, L. B. Rawlings, and C. M. J. Vermeersch. 2010. *Impact Evaluation in Practice*. Washington, DC: World Bank.

Giedion, U., E. Alfonso, and Y. Diaz. 2013. "The Impact of Universal Coverage Schemes in the Developing World: A Systematic Review of the Existing Evidence." Universal Health Coverage Studies Series, UNICO Studies Series 25. World Bank, Washington DC.

Giedion, U., and B. Y. Diaz. 2008. *The Impact of Health Insurance in the Developing World: A Review of the Existing Evidence*. Washington, DC: Brookings Institution Press.

———. 2011. "A Review of the Evidence." In *The Impact of Health Insurance in Low- and Middle-Income Countries*, edited by M.-L. Escobar, 13–32. Washington, DC: Brookings Institution Press.

Giedion, U., B. Y. Diaz, and E. A. Alfonso. 2007. "The Impact of Subsidized Health Insurance on Access, Utilization and Health Status: The Case of Colombia." World Bank, Washington, DC.

Gnawali, D. P., S. Pokhrel, A. Sié, M. Sanon, M. De Allegri, A. Souares, H. Dong, and R. Sauerborn. 2009. "The Effect of Community-Based Health Insurance on the Utilization of Modern Health Care Services: Evidence from Burkina Faso." *Health Policy* 90 (2–3): 214–22.

Gruber, J., N. Hendren, and R. Townsend. 2012. "Demand and Reimbursement Effects of Healthcare Reform: Health Care Utilization and Infant Mortality in Thailand." http://www.nber.org/papers/w17739.

Hou, X., and S. Chao. 2011. "Targeted or Untargeted? The Initial Assessment of a Targeted Health Insurance Program for the Poor in Georgia." *Health Policy* 102 (2–3): 278–85. doi:10.1016/j.healthpol.2011.06.006.

Johar, M. 2009. "The Impact of the Indonesian Health Card Program: A Matching Estimator Approach." *Journal of Health Economics* 28 (1): 35–53. http://www.sciencedirect.com/science/article/pii /S0167629608001331.

Khandker, S. R., G. B. Koolwal, and H. A. Samad. 2009. *Handbook on Impact Evaluation: Quantitative Methods and Practices.* World Bank Training Series. Washington, DC: World Bank.

King, G., E. Gakidou, K. Imai, J. Lakin, R. T. Moore, C. Nall, N. Ravishankar, M. Vargas, M. M. Téllez-Rojo, J. E. Avila, M. H. Avila, and H. H. Llamas. 2009. "Public Policy for the Poor? A Randomised Assessment of the Mexican Universal Health Insurance Programme." *The Lancet* 373 (9673): 1447–54. http://www.sciencedirect.com/science/article/pii /S0140673609602397.

Kraft, A. D., S. A. Quimbo, O. Solon, R. Shimkhada, J. Florentino, and J. W. Peabody. 2009. "The Health and Cost Impact of Care Delay and the Experimental Impact of Insurance on Reducing Delays." *Journal of Pediatrics* 155 (2): 281–85.e1. http://www.sciencedirect.com/science /article/pii/S0022347609001565.

Kutzin, J. 2013. "Health Financing for Universal Coverage and Health System Performance: Concepts and Implications for Policy." *Bulletin of the World Health Organization* 91 (8): 602–11. doi:10.2471/BLT.12.113985.

Lagarde, M., and N. Palmer. 2011. "The Impact of User Fees on Access to Health Services in Low- and Middle-Income Countries." *Cochrane Database of Systematic Reviews* 4 (1).

Lei, X., and W. Lin. 2009. "The New Cooperative Medical Scheme in Rural China: Does More Coverage Mean More Service and Better Health?" *Health Economics* 18 (S2): S25–46. http://dx.doi.org/10.1002/hec.1501.

Levine, D., R. Polimeni, and I. Ramage. 2012. "Insuring Health or Insuring Wealth? An Experimental Evaluation of Health Insurance in Rural Cambodia." *Impact Analyses Series, Ex Post* (08).

Lu, C., B. Chin, G. Li, and C. J. L. Murray. 2009. "Limitations of Methods for Measuring Out-Of-Pocket and Catastrophic Private Health Expenditures." *Bulletin of the World Health Organization* 87: 238–44D. http://www.scielosp.org/scielo.php?script=sci_arttext&pid =S0042-96862009000300019&nrm=iso.

Macinko, J., F. C. Guanais, M. de Fátima, and M. de Souza. 2006. "Evaluation of the Impact of the Family Health Program on Infant Mortality in Brazil, 1990–2002." *Journal of Epidemiology and Community Health* 60 (1): 13–19.

Meyer, C., N. Bellows, M. Campbell, and M. Potts. 2011. *The Impact of Vouchers on the Use and Quality of Health Goods and Services in Developing Countries: A Systematic Review.* London: EPPI-Centre, Social Science Research Unit, Institute of Education, University of London.

Miller, G., D. M. Pinto, and M. Vera-Hernández. 2009. "High-Powered Incentives in Developing Country Health Insurance: Evidence from

Colombia's Régimen Subsidiado." Working Paper 15456, National Bureau of Economic Research. http://www.nber.org/papers/w15456.

Moreno-Serra, R., C. Millett, and P. C. Smith. 2011. "Towards Improved Measurement of Financial Protection in Health." *PLoS Med* 8 (9): e1001087. doi:10.1371/journal.pmed.1001087.

Moreno-Serra, R., and P. C. Smith. 2012. "Does Progress towards Universal Health Coverage Improve Population Health?" *The Lancet* 380 (9845): 917–23. doi:10.1016/S0140-6736(12)61039-3.

Nguyen, C. V. 2012a. "The Impact of Health Insurance for Children: Evidence from Vietnam." Health, Nutrition and Population Working Paper Series 6355. World Bank, Washington DC.

————. 2012b. "The Impact of Voluntary Health Insurance on Health Care Utilization and Out-of-Pocket Payments: New Evidence for Vietnam." *Health Economics* 21 (8): 946–66.

Nguyen, H. T. H., L. Hatt, M. Islam, N. L. Sloan, J. Chowdhury, J.-O. Schmidt, A. Hossain, and H. Wang. 2012. "Encouraging Maternal Health Service Utilization: An Evaluation of the Bangladesh Voucher Program." *Social Science & Medicine* 74 (7): 989–96. doi:10.1016/j.socscimed.2011.11.030.

Panpiemras, J., T. Puttitanun, K. Samphantharak, and K. Thampanishvong. 2011. "Impact of Universal Health Care Coverage on Patient Demand for Health Care Services in Thailand." *Health Policy* 103 (2–3): 228–35. doi:10.1016/j.healthpol.2011.08.008.

Parmar, D., S. Reinhold, A. Souares, G. Savadogo, and R. Sauerborn. 2011. "Does Community-Based Health Insurance Protect Household Assets? Evidence from Rural Africa." *Health Services Research* 47 (2): 819–39. http://dx.doi.org/10.1111/j.1475-6773.2011.01321.x.

Powell-Jackson, T., K. Hanson, C. J. M. Whitty, and E. K. Ansah. 2014. "Who Benefits from Free Healthcare? Evidence from a Randomized Experiment in Ghana." *Journal of Development Economics* 107: 305–19. doi:10.1016/j.jdeveco.2013.11.010.

Quimbo, S. A., J. W. Peabody, R. Shimkhada, J. Florentino, and O. Solon. 2010. "Evidence of a Causal Link between Health Outcomes, Insurance Coverage, and a Policy to Expand Access: Experimental Data from Children in the Philippines." *Health Economics* 20 (5): 620–30. http://dx.doi.org/10.1002/hec.1621.

Rasella, D., R. Aquino, and M. L. Barreto. 2010. "Impact of the Family Health Program on the Quality of Vital Information and Reduction of Child Unattended Deaths in Brazil: An Ecological Longitudinal Study." *BMC Public Health* 10 (1): 380.

Robyn, P. J., G. Fink, A. Sié, and R. Sauerborn. 2012. "Health Insurance and Health-Seeking Behavior: Evidence from a Randomized Community-Based Insurance Rollout in Rural Burkina Faso." *Social Science & Medicine* 75 (4): 595–603. doi:10.1016/j.socscimed.2011.12.018.

Rocha, R., and R. R. Soares. 2010. "Evaluating the Impact of Community -Based Health Interventions: Evidence from Brazil's Family Health Program." *Health Economics* 19 (S1): 126–58.

Ruger, J. P. 2012. "An Alternative Framework for Analyzing Financial Protection in Health." *PLoS Med* 9 (8): e1001294. doi:10.1371/journal. pmed.1001294.

Spaan, E., J. Mathijssen, N. Tromp, F. McBain, A. ten Have, and R. Baltussen. 2012. "The Impact of Health Insurance in Africa and Asia: A Systematic Review." *Bulletin of the World Health Organization* 90 (9): 685–92.

Sparrow, R., A. Suryahadi, and W. Widyanti. 2013. "Social Health Insurance for the Poor: Targeting and Impact of Indonesia's Askeskin Programme." *Social Science & Medicine* 96: 264–71. doi:10.1016/j.socscimed .2012.09.043.

Thornton, R. L., L. E. Hatt, E. M. Field, M. Islam, F. Sol'is Diaz, and M. A. González. 2010. "Social Security Health Insurance for the Informal Sector in Nicaragua: A Randomized Evaluation." *Health Economics* 19 (S1): 181–206. http://Dx.Doi.Org/10.1002/Hec.1635.

Wagstaff, A. 2008. "Measuring Financial Protection in Health." Policy Research Working Paper Series 4554, World Bank, Washington, DC.

———. 2010. "Estimating Health Insurance Impacts under Unobserved Heterogeneity: The Case of Vietnam's Health Care Fund for the Poor." *Health Economics* 19 (2): 189–208. http://dx.doi.org/10.1002/hec.1466.

Wagstaff, A., and M. Pradhan. 2005. "Health Insurance Impacts on Health and Nonmedical Consumption in a Developing Country." Policy Research Working Paper 3563, World Bank, Washington, DC.

Wagstaff, A., and M. Lindelow. 2008. "Can Insurance Increase Financial Risk? The Curious Case of Health Insurance in China." *Journal of Health Economics* 27 (4): 990–1005. doi:10.1016/j.jhealeco.2008.02.002.

Wagstaff, A., M. Lindelow, G. Jun, X. Ling, and Q. Juncheng. 2009. "Extending Health Insurance to the Rural Population: An Impact Evaluation of China's New Cooperative Medical Scheme." *Journal of Health Economics* 28 (1): 1–19. doi:10.1016/j.jhealeco.2008.10.007.

Wagstaff, A., and S. Yu. 2007. "Do Health Sector Reforms Have Their Intended Impacts? The World Bank's Health VIII Project in Gansu Province, China." *Journal of Health Economics* 26 (3): 505–35. doi:10.1016/j.jhealeco.2006.10.006.

Wang, H., W. Yip, L. Zhang, and W. C. Hsiao. 2009. "The Impact of Rural Mutual Health Care on Health Status: Evaluation of a Social Experiment in Rural China." *Health Economics* 18 (S2): S65–82. http://dx.doi. org/10.1002/hec.1465.

White, H. 2009. "Theory-Based Impact Evaluation: Principles and Practice." Working Paper. http://www.3ieimpact.org/admin/pdfs_papers /Working_Paper_3.pdf.

Yip, W., and W. C. Hsiao. 2009. "Non-Evidence-Based Policy: How Effective Is China's New Cooperative Medical Scheme in Reducing Medical Impoverishment?" *Social Science & Medicine* 68 (2): 201–9. http://www.sciencedirect.com/science/article/pii/S0277953608005091.

Yip, W., H. Wang, and W. Hsiao. 2008. "The Impact of Rural Mutual Health Care on Access to Care: Evaluation of a Social Experiment in Rural China." Boston, M.A.: Harvard School of Public Health.

UNICO Questionnaire and Universal Health Coverage Study Series

This appendix can be found online at https://openknowledge.worldbank.org/handle/10986/22011

Index

Boxes, figures, maps, notes, and tables are indicated by *b*, *f*, *m*, *n*, and *t*, respectively.

B

Bangladesh, in literature review, 220,
221, 224
Barros, R., 223
Bellows, B. W., 228
Bellows, N. M., 228
benchmarking financing and
expenditure, 136n2
benefits, 6–8, 30, 67–95
adding services beyond MDG, 69–73,
70–71t
affordability and cost-effectiveness,
80–81, 81b, 86, 96nn3–4
defining explicit packages, 76–79,
77–78t, 94, 169–70, 180
implicit rationing of, 76, 87
key trends in, 7
overall disease burden and, 81,
82t, 95
policy implications, 7–8, 94–95,
188–89, 191
positive and negative lists, 7, 77–79
prioritizing, 68t, 76, 79–86, 81b,
82–85t, 94–95
progressive universalism, alignment
with, 72–73
promised versus effective, 86–90, 95
purchasing and contracting
mechanisms, 90–92, 90t, 91t,
93t, 94
summary packages for UNICO
countries, 74–75t
Beveridge National Health System
model, 169
Bismarck Social Health Insurance
model, 169
Bitran, Ricardo, 50, 53b
bottom-up approach to UHC, 1–2, 4, 27,
28, 35–36, 36f, 48b, 190
Brazil
accreditation of facilities, 151
continuum of care in, 155
empowerment in, 179
enrollment incentives, 45b
expenditure per beneficiary in,
101, 105
explicit benefit package, 170
financing, 207
fiscal transfers, 130
fully tax-financed health
system in, 51
government and external financing,
112, 136n6
health care providers in, 143–44, 145
ID system, 43
identifying and targeting poor and
vulnerable populations, 41b,
41f, 48b
implicit rationing in, 87
informal sector coverage in, 54

information systems in, 177
life expectancy/mortality, 205
in literature review, 223–24, 227
macroeconomic indicators, 203
merger of MOH and SHI in, 37
output-based payment, 174
poverty and informal sector
population ratios, 54, 55f
private provider participation in, 147
purchaser-provider split, 168
purchasing and contracting for
benefits, 92
risk pooling, 127
sociodemographic indicators, 198
subnational delegation of
responsibilities in, 171
Burkina Faso, in literature review, 220,
222, 225

C

Camacho, A., 227
Camacho, Adriana, 50
Cambodia, in literature review, 224,
225, 226
Canada, primary care outpatient
coverage in, 88
capitation, 44, 87, 92, 94, 96n9, 129,
130, 146, 172, 173, 174–75
case-based payment methods, 92
CBHI (community-based health
insurance) programs, 220–21,
222, 228, 229
CCTs (conditional cash transfers), 41b,
45b, 242n1
Celhay, P., 219, 221
centralized versus decentralized health
systems, 128–29, 129t, 170–72
Chen, Y., 226
child health
benefits, 69, 71t, 72, 73, 76
coverage, 38, 50
elimination of cost-sharing for, 9
financing and expenditure, 101, 105,
119, 120, 127
improving provision of, 143
mortality rates, 204, 206t, 207, 208f
programs limited to, 10
Chile
accreditation of facilities, 151
AUGE (Explicit Health Guarantees)
law, 9, 132, 169–70
continuum of care in, 155
cost-sharing, 120b
coverage, 212
democratization levels, 198
earmarking, 116–17
empowerment in, 179, 180
expenditure per beneficiary in, 101,
103, 106
fiscal transfers, 129

Environmental Benefits Statement

The World Bank Group is committed to reducing its environmental footprint. In support of this commitment, the Publishing and Knowledge Division leverages electronic publishing options and print-on-demand technology, which is located in regional hubs worldwide. Together, these initiatives enable print runs to be lowered and shipping distances decreased, resulting in reduced paper consumption, chemical use, greenhouse gas emissions, and waste.

The Publishing and Knowledge Division follows the recommended standards for paper use set by the Green Press Initiative. Whenever possible, books are printed on 50 percent to 100 percent postconsumer recycled paper, and at least 50 percent of the fiber in our book paper is either unbleached or bleached using Totally Chlorine Free (TCF), Processed Chlorine Free (PCF), or Enhanced Elemental Chlorine Free (EECF) processes.

More information about the Bank's environmental philosophy can be found at http://crinfo.worldbank.org/wbcrinfo/node/4.

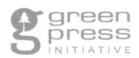